# Juicing to manage diabetes

*A Natural Approach to Managing Diabetes*

**Kai Norris**

# Copyright © 2023 **Kai Norris**

All rights reserved. No part of this book may be reproduced or transmitted in any form or by any means, electronic or mechanical, including photocopying, recording, or by any information

storage and retrieval system. Without permission in writing from the author.

This book is a work of non-fiction. The views expressed are solely those of the author and do not necessarily reflect the views of the publisher, and the publisher hereby disclaims any responsibility for them.

# TABLE OF CONTENT

# INTRODUCTION

Diabetes is a very deadly disease that affects millions of people worldwide. It is distinguished by elevated glucose levels in the blood, which can lead to a variety of complications over time. While conventional treatments for diabetes include medication and dietary changes, many people are turning to natural remedies to help them manage their condition.

Juicing is one such cure. Juicing is the process of extracting juice from fruits and vegetables, and it can be a quick and easy way to consume a variety of nutrients in concentrated form. Some people believe that juicing can help with diabetes management because certain fruits and vegetables have been shown to lower blood sugar levels.

It is important to note, however, that juicing is not a replacement for medical treatment. Before making any changes to their diabetes treatment plan, diabetics should always consult with their healthcare provider. Furthermore, some fruits and vegetables may contain high levels of natural sugars, which can cause blood sugar levels to spike. As a result, it's critical to select the right ingredients and carefully monitor blood sugar levels.

Despite these factors, juicing can be an effective addition to a diabetes management plan when combined with other healthy lifestyle changes. In this article, we'll look at the potential benefits of juicing for diabetes, as well as the best fruits and vegetables to include in a diabetes-friendly juice and some juicing safety and effectiveness tips. Juicing is the process of extracting juice from fruits and vegetables, which is frequently done with the aid of a juicer. Juicing can provide a concentrated source of nutrients such as vitamins, minerals, and antioxidants, which can aid in overall health.

Certain juices may have properties that can help regulate blood sugar levels and improve insulin sensitivity in the case of diabetes. Individuals with diabetes may be able to better manage their condition and reduce their reliance on medication by including fresh juices in their diet. It is important to note, however, that juicing should not be used in place of medical treatment or dietary recommendations from a healthcare professional.

In this article, we will look at the benefits of juicing for diabetes management, as well as the best fruits and vegetables to juice and how to incorporate juicing into a diabetic diet. Juicing, however, should not be used as a sole treatment for diabetes, and individuals should always consult with their healthcare provider before incorporating juicing into their treatment plan. It is critical to consume low-sugar fruits and vegetables to avoid blood sugar spikes. Overall, juicing can be a useful addition to a comprehensive diabetes management plan because it provides a tasty and nutrient-dense way to increase important vitamins and minerals in the diet.

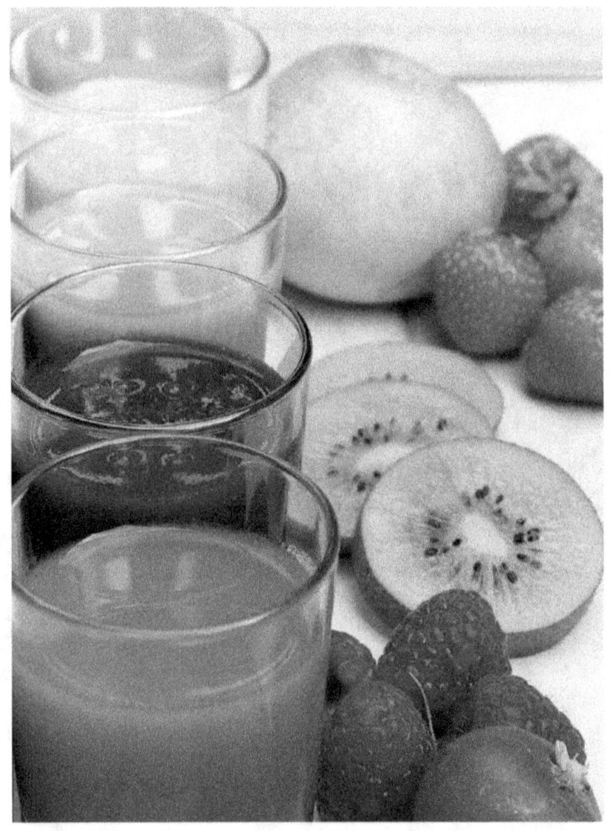

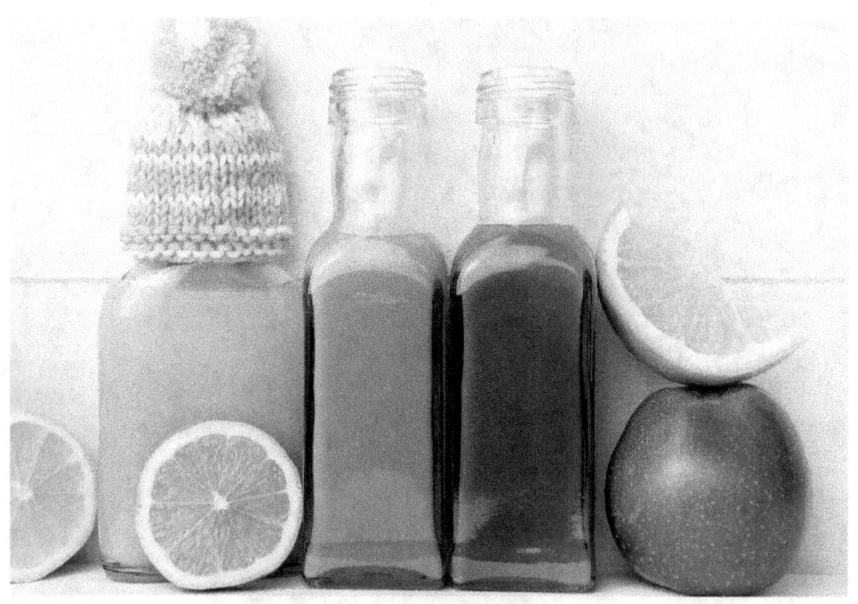

# CHAPTER ONE

## Diabetes and Nutrition: An Overview

Diabetes is a deadly disease that affects millions of people around the world. It is characterized by high blood sugar levels, which can lead to a variety of health problems if left untreated. While there is no cure for diabetes, proper nutrition can help manage the condition and reduce the risk of complications. In this overview, we will look at the relationship between diabetes and nutrition and how people with diabetes can make healthy food choices to stay healthy.

Maintaining healthy blood sugar levels is one of the most important aspects of diabetes management. This can be accomplished by eating a varied diet rich in nutrients.

Carbohydrates, in particular, have a significant impact on blood sugar levels, and diabetics must be mindful of the types and amounts of carbs they consume. Foods high in refined carbohydrates, such as white bread, pasta, and sugary snacks, can cause blood sugar levels to spike.

Individuals with diabetes should instead focus on consuming complex carbohydrates that are high in fiber, such as whole grains, fruits, and vegetables.

Protein is also an important component of a healthy diabetes diet. It helps to maintain muscle mass and can help to slow carbohydrate absorption, which can help to stabilize blood sugar levels. Individuals with diabetes should eat lean protein sources such as poultry, fish, tofu, and legumes.

It is critical to limit your consumption of red and processed meats, as they have been linked to an increased risk of heart disease and other health problems.

Fat consumption is another important aspect of diabetes nutrition. While fats are an important part of a healthy diet, people with diabetes must be mindful of the types of fats they consume. Saturated and trans fats, which are found in foods such as butter, red meat, and processed snacks, can raise cholesterol levels and increase the risk of heart disease.

Individuals with diabetes should instead focus on eating unsaturated fats, which can be found in foods like nuts, seeds, and oily fish.

Individuals with diabetes should pay attention to their intake of micronutrients such as vitamins and minerals, in addition to macronutrients such as carbohydrates,

protein, and fat. Certain vitamins and minerals, such as magnesium, chromium, and vitamin D, can help with blood sugar control. Eating a variety of whole foods, such as fruits, vegetables, nuts, and seeds, can help ensure that people with diabetes get the nutrients they need to stay healthy.

Individuals with diabetes should also be mindful of their portion sizes and overall calorie intake. While eating healthy foods is important, eating too much of anything can lead to weight gain, making blood sugar management more difficult. Working with a registered dietitian can be beneficial in developing a meal plan that meets an individual's nutritional needs while also supporting their overall health and wellness.

The glycemic index measures how quickly carbohydrates in a food raise blood glucose levels. High glycemic index foods, such as white bread and sugary drinks, can cause blood sugar levels to spike quickly. Individuals with diabetes can help maintain stable blood sugar levels by eating foods with a lower glycemic index, such as whole grains and non-starchy vegetables.

Sugar substitutes like stevia and Splenda can be a useful tool for diabetics who want to enjoy sweet foods without raising their blood sugar levels. However, it is critical to use sugar substitutes sparingly and to maintain an overall balanced and nutrient-rich diet.

Individuals with diabetes should consume alcohol in moderation because it can affect blood sugar levels. Drinking alcohol on an empty stomach can cause blood sugar levels to drop dangerously low, whereas drinking alcohol with a meal can cause blood sugar levels to rise dangerously high. Individuals with diabetes should closely monitor their blood sugar levels when consuming alcohol and limit their intake to one drink per day for women and two drinks per day for men.

Regular physical activity can also aid in diabetes management by increasing insulin sensitivity and lowering the risk of complications. Diabetes patients should aim to incorporate both aerobic exercise, such as brisk walking or cycling, and strength training into their daily routine.

In addition to diet and exercise, stress management and adequate sleep are critical components of diabetes management. Stress can raise blood sugar levels and make managing the condition more difficult, while a lack of sleep can impair insulin sensitivity and glucose metabolism.

Individuals with diabetes can benefit from prioritizing self-care activities such as meditation or yoga, as well as aiming for seven to eight hours of sleep per night.

Individuals with diabetes can improve their quality of life and reduce their risk of complications by taking a holistic approach to diabetes management that includes proper nutrition, regular exercise, stress management, and adequate sleep. To develop a personalized diabetes management plan that meets individual needs and goals, it is critical to collaborate closely with a healthcare team that includes a registered dietitian and a physician.

Diabetes and nutrition are inextricably linked and making positive dietary and lifestyle changes can have a significant impact on diabetes management and overall health. Individuals with diabetes can improve their overall health and well-being by working with a healthcare professional to develop a personalized nutrition plan that meets their specific needs and goals. Aside from the factors and dietary patterns mentioned above, certain foods and nutrients may have specific benefits for people with diabetes. These are some examples:

**Berries**: Berries rich in antioxidants and fiber, such as blueberries, raspberries, and strawberries, have been shown to help regulate blood sugar levels.

**Cinnamon:** Studies have shown that cinnamon improves insulin sensitivity and lowers blood sugar levels.

Magnesium is an essential mineral that is involved in many bodily processes, including glucose metabolism. Some research suggests that taking magnesium supplements may help improve insulin sensitivity and blood sugar control.

**Omega-3 fatty acids**: Omega-3 fatty acids, which are found in fatty fish like salmon and sardines, have been shown to improve insulin sensitivity and decrease inflammation in the body.

**Vinegar:** According to some studies, vinegar can help lower blood sugar levels and improve insulin sensitivity.

While these foods and nutrients may have specific benefits for people with diabetes, they should still be consumed as part of a well-balanced and varied diet.

Individuals with diabetes can benefit from learning more about food labels, meal planning, and healthy cooking techniques in addition to working with a healthcare professional to develop a personalized nutrition plan. Individuals with diabetes can improve their overall health and reduce their risk of complications by making small, sustainable changes to their diet and lifestyle. Physical activity is also essential in diabetes management. Regular exercise can help improve insulin sensitivity and blood sugar control while also lowering the risk of complications like heart disease and stroke.

Individuals with diabetes should also monitor their blood sugar levels on a regular basis and work closely with a healthcare professional to adjust their treatment plan as needed. Changes in medication, insulin dosage, or other treatments may be included. To summarize, diabetes and nutrition are inextricably linked, and making positive dietary and lifestyle changes can have a significant impact on diabetes management and overall health. Individuals with diabetes can improve their quality of life and lower their risk of complications by working with a healthcare professional to develop a personalized treatment plan that includes diet, exercise, stress management, and medication as needed.

Individuals with diabetes must choose activities that are both safe and appropriate for their condition. A healthcare professional can assist in developing an exercise plan that takes an individual's age, fitness level, and any other medical conditions into account. Another important aspect of diabetes management is stress management, as stress can cause blood sugar levels to fluctuate, making it more difficult to manage the condition. Deep breathing, meditation, and yoga are all techniques that can help to reduce stress and improve overall well-being.

To summarize, proper nutrition is a critical component of diabetes management. Individuals with diabetes can maintain healthy blood sugar levels and lower their risk of complications by focusing on a balanced diet that includes a variety of nutrient-rich foods. Individuals with diabetes have the power to take control of their health and live their best life, whether with the help of a registered dietitian or by making simple changes to their diet and lifestyle.

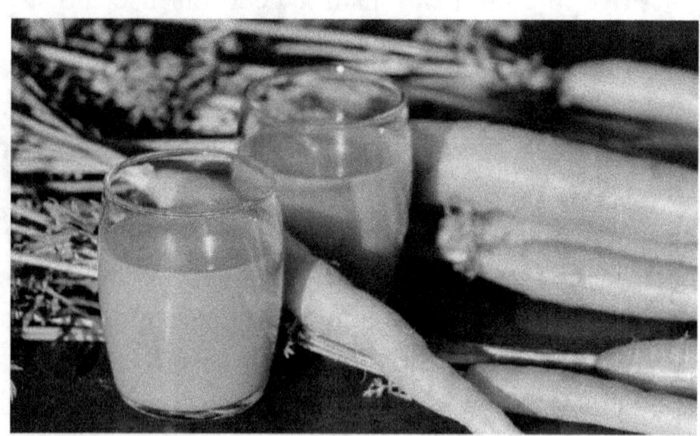

# CHAPTER TWO

## Juicing for Diabetes: Benefits and Risks

Juicing for diabetes is a hotly debated topic. While some people believe that juicing is an effective way to manage diabetes, others argue that it is risky and even harmful. In this article, we will look at the benefits and risks of juicing for diabetes and help you make an informed decision about whether it is right for you.

Let's start with the benefits of juicing for diabetes. One of the most significant advantages is that it can help you increase your intake of fruits and vegetables, which are essential for diabetes management. Fruits and vegetables are high in vitamins, minerals, and antioxidants, which can help regulate blood sugar levels, boost the immune system, and lower the risk of complications like heart disease and stroke.

Juicing can also help you get more fiber, which is an important nutrient for diabetes management. Fiber helps to regulate blood sugar levels by slowing the absorption of glucose in the body. It can also help you feel full, which can help you avoid overeating and maintain a healthy weight.

Another advantage of juicing for diabetes is that it can be a quick and easy way to consume a variety of fruits and vegetables. Many people struggle to get enough fruits and vegetables in their diet, but juicing can help.

However, it is also important to be aware of the risks of juicing for diabetes. One of the main risks is that juicing can cause a rapid spike in blood sugar levels, especially if you juice sugary fruits. As a result, it is critical to select fruits and vegetables that are low in sugar and high in fiber, such as leafy greens, cucumber, and celery.

The risk of juicing for diabetes is nutrient imbalance. When you juice fruits and vegetables, you remove the fiber and some of the nutrients found in the skin and pulp. This can result in a nutrient imbalance in the body, especially if you rely heavily on juicing as your primary source of fruits and vegetables.

When juicing fruits and vegetables, there is the possibility of contamination. If you do not wash and prepare your product properly, you may consume harmful bacteria or chemicals. Juicing for diabetes can be a useful addition to your diabetes management plan, but it should not be used in place of healthy eating habits, regular exercise, and medication.

If you're thinking about juicing, talk to your doctor or a registered dietitian first to make sure it's safe for you and won't interfere with any medications or treatments you're taking.

It is critical to choose fruits and vegetables with low glycemic index values when juicing. Foods with a high glycemic index can cause a rapid spike in blood sugar levels, which can be dangerous for diabetics. Low glycemic index fruits and vegetables include leafy greens, cucumbers, celery, and broccoli. When juicing for diabetes, it is also critical to regularly monitor your blood sugar levels. Juicing can cause a rapid increase in blood sugar levels, especially if you juice sugary fruits.

If you notice that your blood sugar levels are higher than usual after juicing, you may need to adjust your juicing recipe or reduce the amount of fruit in your juice. When juicing, it is critical to use a high-quality juicer that can extract as much juice as possible while preserving the nutrients. Cold-pressed juicers are popular because they extract juice with gentle pressure rather than heat, which can destroy some of the nutrients. When purchasing pre-made juices from stores or juice bars, exercise caution. Many of these juices contain added sugars or are made from fruits with a high glycemic index, which can be harmful to diabetics.

It is always best to make your own juice at home from fresh, whole fruits and vegetables. Juicing for diabetes can be a healthy and delicious way to increase your intake of fruits and vegetables, but it is important to understand the risks and benefits. Consult your healthcare provider and a registered dietitian to determine if juicing is right for you and to develop a safe and effective juicing plan. When juicing for diabetes, it is critical to pay attention to portion sizes in addition to monitoring blood sugar levels and selecting the right fruits and vegetables to juice.

A single serving of juice is typically 4-6 ounces, which is much smaller than a typical glass of juice. Too much juice can cause a rapid rise in blood sugar levels, so stick to small portions and avoid using juice as a meal replacement. To reap the most benefits from diabetes juicing, include a variety of fruits and vegetables in your recipes. This can help ensure that you are getting a variety of nutrients, such as vitamins, minerals, and antioxidants. Kale, spinach, cucumber, celery, ginger, and lemon are all popular diabetes-friendly juice ingredients.

Another important factor to consider when juicing for diabetes is the timing of your juice consumption. It is best to consume juice in the morning or early afternoon when your body is most capable of processing the sugar and nutrients. Drinking juice in the evening or before bed can disrupt your sleep and cause blood sugar levels to spike during the night.

Overall, juicing for diabetes can be a beneficial addition to your diabetes management plan, but it is important to proceed with caution and to consult with your healthcare provider and a registered dietitian before beginning. Juicing, with the right guidance and a balanced approach, can help you increase your intake of fruits and vegetables while also managing your diabetes more effectively.

One of the primary advantages of juicing for diabetes is that it can help you increase your intake of fruits and vegetables. Many people with diabetes do not consume enough fruits and vegetables, making it difficult to meet their nutrient requirements and maintain healthy blood sugar levels. Juicing can be a convenient and tasty way to increase your intake of these nutrient-dense foods.

Fruits and vegetables are an important part of a diabetic's diet because they are low in calories and high in fiber, vitamins, minerals, and antioxidants. Vitamins and minerals are essential for overall health and well-being, and antioxidants can help protect against the damage caused by oxidative stress, which is a common complication of diabetes. Juicing can also help you manage your diabetes more effectively by providing a quick and easy source of nutrition. Juice made from diabetes-friendly fruits and vegetables can help stabilize your blood sugar levels, boost your energy, and improve your overall health. Juicing can also be beneficial for people who have difficulty chewing or digesting whole fruits and vegetables.

Another advantage of juicing for diabetes is that it can be a fun and creative way to experiment with different flavors and ingredients. There are countless juice recipes available online and in cookbooks, so you can easily find recipes that suit your taste preferences and nutritional requirements. You can also add herbs, spices, and plant-based protein powders to your juices to make them your own.

Furthermore, juicing can be a useful tool for people with diabetes who want to increase their intake of fruits and vegetables while also managing their blood sugar levels more effectively. However, it is important to proceed with caution and to consult with your healthcare provider and a registered dietitian before beginning. With the right guidance and a balanced approach, juicing can be a delicious and nutritious addition to your diabetes management plan. One potential benefit of juicing for diabetes is that it can be a more appealing way to consume bitter or less appealing vegetables.

Many vegetables that are highly recommended for diabetics, such as kale, spinach, and bitter melon, can be difficult to eat raw or cooked. Juicing these vegetables with sweeter fruits like apples, pears, or berries can make them more enjoyable to consume while retaining their nutritional benefits.

Another advantage of juicing is that it can help you get more hydration in your diet. Drinking enough fluids is important for diabetics because high blood sugar levels can cause increased urination and dehydration. Juicing can help you stay hydrated while also providing important nutrients and antioxidants.

Another risk is that some fruits and vegetables, such as carrots, beets, and pineapples, are high in natural sugars, which can cause blood sugar levels to spike. It is critical to use these ingredients sparingly or to balance them out with low-sugar fruits and vegetables such as cucumbers, celery, or leafy greens.

It is important to note that juicing should not be used as a substitute for a healthy, balanced diet that includes whole foods. While juicing can be a convenient and tasty way to consume fruits and vegetables, it is also important to eat a variety of whole foods to ensure that you are getting everything of the nutrients you want.

In conclusion, juicing can provide several benefits for people with diabetes, including increased intake of fruits and vegetables, hydration, and a more palatable way to consume bitter or less appealing vegetables. However, it is critical to be aware of the potential risks and to use juicing as part of a balanced and healthy diet.

Consult your healthcare provider and a registered dietitian to determine if juicing is right for you and to develop a safe and effective juicing plan. When incorporating juicing into your diabetes treatment plan, it is also important to consider the juicer's quality and the juicing process.

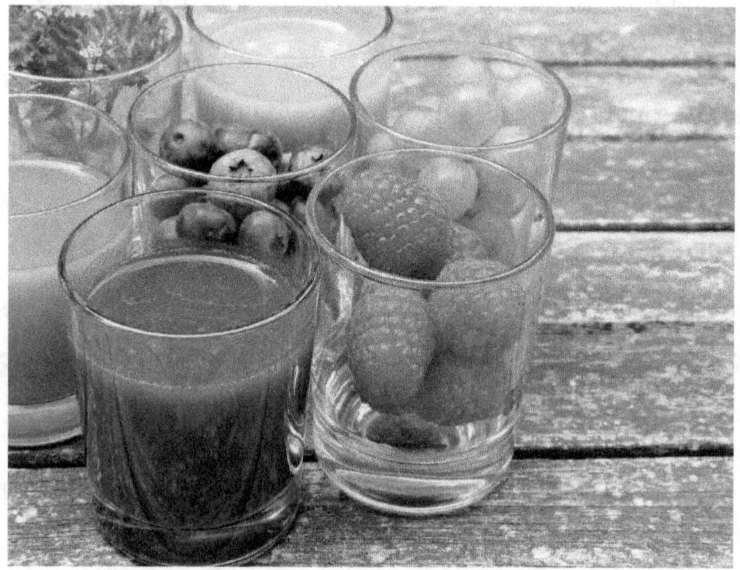

# CHAPTER THREE

## Essential Nutrients for Managing Diabetes

Diabetes management requires proper nutrition, which includes eating foods that contain essential nutrients that help control blood sugar levels. Here are some essential nutrients that can help with diabetes management:

**Fiber**: Fiber is an important nutrient for diabetes management. It reduces glucose absorption in the bloodstream, preventing blood sugar spikes. High-fiber foods also keep you fuller for longer, reducing your desire to snack on unhealthy foods. Whole grains, fruits, vegetables, beans, and nuts are examples of high-fiber foods.

**Protein**: Protein is required for the formation and repair of tissues in the body. It also helps you feel fuller for longer and slows glucose absorption. Is good to go for lean proteins like chicken, fish, tofu, and legumes.

**Healthy Fats**: Omega-3 fatty acids, for example, can help reduce inflammation and improve insulin sensitivity. Avocados, nuts, seeds, and fatty fish like salmon are all examples of healthy fats.

**Vitamins and minerals**: Vitamins and minerals are necessary for overall health and well-being. Vitamin D, vitamin B12, magnesium, and potassium are among the most important vitamins and minerals for diabetes management.

**Water**: Getting enough water is essential for diabetes management. It aids in the removal of excess sugar and keeps you hydrated, both of which are essential for overall health.

**Chromium**: is a mineral that aids in insulin metabolism, thereby improving insulin sensitivity and glucose tolerance. Broccoli, grape juice, and whole grains are all high in chromium.

**Zinc**: is yet another mineral required for insulin production and glucose metabolism. Oysters, lean meats, beans, and nuts are all high in zinc.

**Magnesium:** is a mineral that is essential for glucose metabolism and insulin sensitivity. Low magnesium levels have been linked to an increased risk of developing type 2 diabetes. Leafy green vegetables, nuts, seeds, and whole grains are all high in magnesium.

Probiotics are live bacteria that can help improve gut health and reduce inflammation, which is important for diabetes management. Probiotics may also improve insulin sensitivity and glucose tolerance, according to some research.

Resistant starch is a type of carbohydrate that resists digestion in the small intestine and instead passes through to the large intestine where it acts as a prebiotic, feeding beneficial gut bacteria. It has been demonstrated that resistant starch improves insulin sensitivity and lowers blood sugar levels. Green bananas cooked and cooled potatoes, and legumes are all good sources of resistant starch.

**Polyphenols** are antioxidants found in plant foods that have been shown to have anti-inflammatory and anti-diabetic properties. Polyphenols may improve insulin sensitivity, lower blood sugar levels, and prevent diabetic complications, according to some research. Berries, tea, cocoa, and spices like cinnamon and turmeric are high in polyphenols.

**Coenzyme Q10** is a powerful antioxidant that is involved in the production of cellular energy. According to some research, CoQ10 may improve insulin sensitivity and lower the risk of diabetic complications. Fatty fish, organ meats, and nuts are all high in CoQ10. Vitamin C: As an antioxidant, vitamin C can help reduce inflammation and improve insulin sensitivity. Citrus fruits, berries, kiwi, and bell peppers are all high in vitamin C.

**Vitamin E**: Another antioxidant that can help reduce inflammation and improve insulin sensitivity is vitamin E. Nuts, seeds, and leafy green vegetables are high in vitamin E.

B vitamins, specifically B6, B12, and folate, are essential for maintaining healthy blood sugar levels. Whole grains, leafy green vegetables, and fortified cereals are all good sources of B vitamins.

**Phytochemicals**: Phytochemicals are naturally occurring plant compounds with anti-inflammatory and anti-diabetic properties. Flavonoids and anthocyanins, for example, may improve insulin sensitivity and lower the risk of diabetic complications. Brightly colored fruits and vegetables, such as berries, cherries, spinach, and kale, are high in phytochemicals.

**L-Carnitine:** L-carnitine is an amino acid that aids in the metabolism of energy. According to some studies, L-carnitine may improve insulin sensitivity and lower blood sugar levels. Red meat, fish, and dairy products are all good sources of L-carnitine.

**Alpha-lipoic acid:** is a powerful antioxidant that has been shown to improve insulin sensitivity and reduce oxidative stress, both of which are factors in diabetic complications. Spinach, broccoli, and organ meats are high in alpha-lipoic acid.

**Selenium**: is a mineral that aids in antioxidant function and immune system function. According to some research, selenium may improve insulin sensitivity and lower the risk of diabetic complications. Brazil nuts, seafood, and whole grains are all high in selenium.

**Vitamin K**: is a fat-soluble vitamin that promotes blood clotting and bone health. According to some research, vitamin K may improve insulin sensitivity and lower the risk of diabetes-related complications. Leafy green vegetables like spinach, kale, and broccoli are high in vitamin K.

It is important to note that, while these essential nutrients may help with diabetes management, they are not a replacement for medical treatment or medication management. Working with your healthcare provider to develop a personalized diabetes management plan that includes regular physical activity, stress management, and medication management, as needed, in addition to a healthy diet rich in essential nutrients is critical.

Work with your healthcare provider to develop a personalized diabetes management plan that takes your specific nutritional needs and medical history into account. Regular blood sugar monitoring, as well as regular check-ins with your healthcare provider, can help ensure that your diabetes is managed effectively.

People with diabetes can live long, healthy lives and reduce their risk of diabetes-related complications by making lifestyle changes such as eating a healthy diet, staying physically active, and managing stress.

Finally, managing diabetes necessitates a multifaceted approach that includes proper nutrition and lifestyle changes. Making sure your body gets all of the nutrients it requires is an important part of diabetes management. People with diabetes can improve their blood sugar control and overall health by eating foods high in fiber, omega-3s, magnesium, vitamin D, chromium, vitamin C, and B vitamins. To develop a personalized diabetes nutrition plan, it is always recommended to consult with a healthcare professional or registered dietitian.

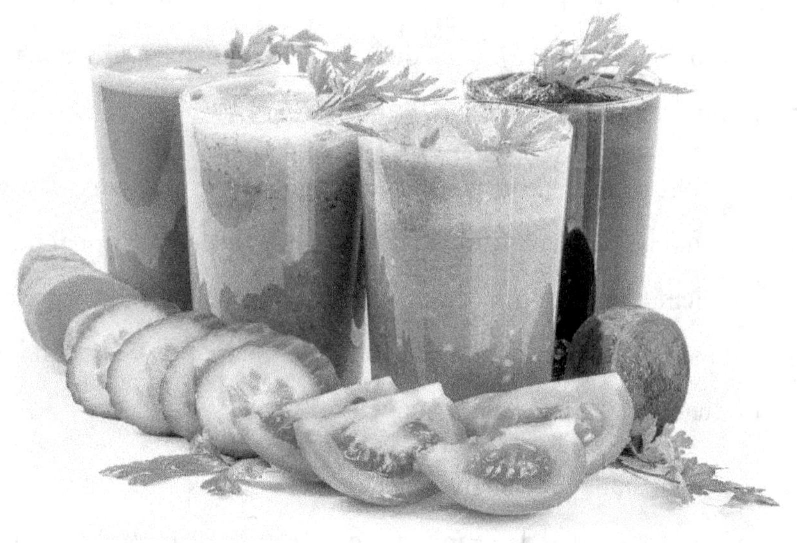

# CHAPTER FOUR

## Top 5 Juicing Recipes for Diabetes

Juicing can be a great way to get more nutrients into your diet, especially if you have diabetes. Here are five top juicing recipes that are diabetes-friendly:

**1. Apple, Carrot, and Ginger Juice**: This delicious and nutritious juice recipe is ideal for diabetics. The combination of ingredients aids in blood sugar regulation while also providing essential vitamins and minerals.

Ingredients:

2 cored and chopped apples 2 peeled and chopped carrots 2 teaspoons freshly grated ginger 1/2 cup water

Instructions:

1. In a blender, combine the apples, carrots, and ginger and blend until smooth.

2. Add the water and blend for 30 seconds more.

3. Pass the mixture through a fine mesh sieve to remove the solids.

4. Strain the juice into a glass and serve.

This juice is high in vitamins and minerals, which are beneficial for diabetics. Apples and carrots are both high in fiber, which aids in blood sugar regulation. Ginger reduces inflammation and aids digestion. This juice is also low in calories and sugar, making it an excellent choice for those trying to keep a healthy weight.

**2. Beet and spinach juice:** Beet juice is high in antioxidants and is known to reduce inflammation. It also contains a lot of vitamins and minerals when combined with spinach.

- 2 large peeled and chopped beets - 4 cups fresh spinach - 2 cored and chopped apples - 2 carrots - 1/2 inch peeled and chopped ginger - 1/4 cup fresh lemon juice

Instructions:

1. Combine all of the ingredients in a blender and blend until smooth..

2. Strain the juice through a fine-mesh strainer, pressing the solids down with a spoon or spatula to extract as much juice as possible.

3. Serve the juice immediately or refrigerate in an airtight container for up to 5 days.

Explanation: Beet and spinach juice is a tasty and nutritious drink that may be beneficial to diabetics. Beets are high in fiber, which aids in blood sugar regulation, whereas spinach is high in antioxidants, which help reduce inflammation and protect against oxidative stress.

Apples and carrots add vitamins and minerals, while ginger and lemon give it a zesty flavor. This juice is simple to make and can be kept in the fridge for up to 5 days. Enjoy this drink as a healthy snack or as part of a meal.

**3. Cucumber and celery juice**: This juice is high in potassium, which is important for blood sugar control. Cucumber and celery are a delicious and refreshing combination.

Cucumber and celery juice can help with diabetes.

Ingredients:

• 1 large peeled and chopped cucumber • 2 large celery stalks chopped • 1/2 lemon juiced • 1/4 teaspoon sea salt • 1 cup water

Instructions:

1. In a blender, combine the cucumber, celery, lemon, and sea salt.

2. Puree the ingredients until smooth.

3. Blend in the water until all of the ingredients are combined.

4. Pass the juice through a fine mesh sieve to strain it.

5. Serve immediately or store in an airtight container in the fridge for up to two days.

Cucumber and Celery Juice Benefits for Diabetes: Cucumber and celery juice is a nutritious drink that can assist people with diabetes in managing their blood sugar levels.

Cucumber and celery's high water content aids in the removal of toxins from the body, which can aid in the regulation of blood sugar levels. Lemon juice and sea salt can also help to improve digestion, which can aid in diabetes management. Cucumber and celery also contain important vitamins and minerals that can help boost the immune system.

**4. Carrot and Orange Juice:** Carrot juice is beneficial to diabetics because it regulates blood sugar levels and is high in vitamins and minerals. Orange juice adds a tasty and sweet flavor to the mix. This recipe is an excellent source of vitamins and minerals that are especially beneficial to diabetics. Carrots are high in beta-carotene, which aids the body's sugar processing, and oranges are high in vitamin C, which aids iron absorption.

Ingredients:

2 cups cold water - 2 large carrots, peeled and roughly chopped - 2 oranges, peeled and roughly chopped

Instructions:

1. In a blender, combine the carrots and oranges and blend on high until smooth.

2. Add the water and blend until all of the ingredients are combined.

3. Strain the mixture through a fine-mesh sieve, pressing on the solids as much as possible to extract as much juice as possible.

4. Pour the juice into a chilled glass and enjoy!

This recipe can be tailored to individual preferences by including additional ingredients such as lemon, apples, ginger, or honey. It is best to avoid adding added sugars to juice if you have diabetes.

**5. Pineapple and Kale Juice**: Pineapple is beneficial to diabetics because it reduces inflammation and regulates blood sugar levels. Because kale is high in vitamins and minerals, this juice is an excellent choice for diabetics.

Diabetes and Pineapple Kale Juice:

Ingredients:

- 2 cups chopped fresh pineapple - 2 cups washed and chopped kale
- 1 small cucumber, peeled and chopped - 2 stalks celery, chopped

- 1 chopped large carrot

- 1-inch piece peeled and grated ginger - 1/2 cup water

- 1 lime juice

Instructions:

1. In a blender, put all together with the ingredients and blend until smooth.

2. Remove any pulp from the juice by straining it through a fine mesh strainer.

3. Pour the juice into glasses and serve right away.

This Pineapple Kale Juice is excellent for diabetes management. Bromelain, a compound found in pineapple, helps to reduce inflammation and regulate blood sugar levels. Kale is also high in fiber, which slows the absorption of sugar into the bloodstream. Cucumbers celery, carrot, and ginger all contribute nutrients and flavor to the juice. The lime juice gives the drink a tart flavor and helps to regulate blood sugar levels. To help manage diabetes and stay healthy, drink this delicious and nutritious juice. In addition to aiding in diabetes management, this juice is high in vitamins and minerals, making it an excellent addition to any diet.

How much juice should a diabetic drink on a daily basis? The amount of juice a diabetic should drink on a daily basis is determined by a number of factors, including their overall health, blood sugar levels, and dietary preferences. However, because of its high sugar content, it is generally recommended that people with diabetes limit their intake of fruit juice.

Fruit juice can quickly raise blood sugar levels, resulting in dangerous spikes and crashes for diabetics. A serving of fruit juice is typically defined as 4 ounces or half a cup. In general, people with diabetes should limit their fruit juice consumption to no more than one serving per day.

It is critical for people with diabetes to consume whole fruits rather than fruit juice. Whole fruits have more fiber, which slows sugar absorption into the bloodstream and can help regulate blood sugar levels. Furthermore, whole fruits contain more nutrients and are more filling than fruit juice, which can aid in weight management and overall health.

If you have specific questions or concerns about your diabetes diet, speak with a registered dietitian or healthcare provider who can provide personalized guidance and recommendations.

If you must drink fruit juice, it is best to choose 100% juice with no added sugars or artificial sweeteners.

Consider diluting your fruit juice with water to reduce the overall sugar content and impact on blood sugar levels.

Remember that juice isn't the only source of sugar in your diet. Sugar can also be found in candy, soda, baked goods, and processed foods, so it's important to keep track of your total sugar intake and limit added sugars as much as possible.

Some vegetable juices, such as tomato or carrot juice, may contain less sugar than fruit juice and thus be a healthier option for diabetics.

When making dietary choices, keep your personal needs and preferences in mind. Some diabetics may be able to tolerate more fruit juice than others, while others may choose to avoid it entirely. A healthcare provider or registered dietitian can assist you in determining what is best for your specific situation.

Finally, it's critical to regularly monitor your blood sugar levels and adjust your diet based on the results. Keeping track of your blood sugar levels can help you identify patterns and make informed food and beverage choices.

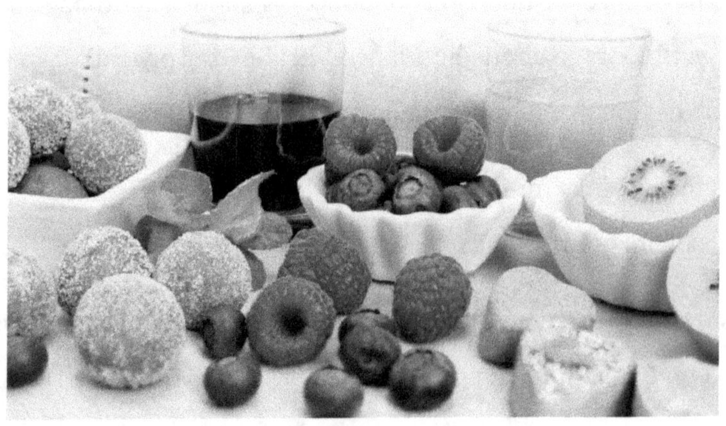

# CHAPTER FIVE

## Best Fruits and Vegetables for Juicing with Diabetes

**Fruits:**

1. Apples

2. Blueberries

3. Strawberries

4. Oranges Fruits:

5. Grapefruit

6. Pineapple

7. Cranberries

**Vegetables:**

1. Spinach

2. Kale

3. Celery

4. Cucumbers

5. Carrots

6. Beets

7. Broccoli

8. Peppers

Certain fruits and vegetables can be beneficial when it comes to juicing and diabetes. Fruits and vegetables high in fiber, vitamins, minerals, and antioxidants are especially beneficial for blood sugar control. Juicing these fruits and vegetables can help you lose weight and lower your risk of developing Type 2 diabetes.

Apples, oranges, grapefruits, lemons, limes, and blueberries are the best fruits for juicing with diabetes. These fruits contain essential vitamins, minerals, and antioxidants that can aid in blood sugar regulation. Apples are particularly beneficial because they contain pectin, a natural fiber that helps slow sugar absorption into the bloodstream. Oranges and grapefruits are high in fiber and vitamin C as well.

Kale, spinach, celery, cucumbers, and beets are among the vegetables that are beneficial for juicing with diabetes. These veggies are low in sugar and high in vitamins, minerals, and antioxidants. Kale and spinach are high in vitamin A, which aids in insulin production regulation.

Lutein, found in celery, helps to protect cells from damage caused by high blood sugar levels. Cucumbers are high in vitamin K, which aids in blood clotting regulation. Be Juicing fruits and vegetables provides a concentrated dose of vitamins, minerals, and other essential nutrients. Juicing can help diabetics stabilize their blood sugar levels, reduce inflammation, and improve their overall health.

Leafy greens like kale, spinach, and Swiss chard, which are high in fiber, vitamins, and minerals, are among the best fruits and vegetables for juicing with diabetes. Other diabetes-friendly fruits and vegetables include apples, oranges, carrots, tomatoes, beets, celery, cucumbers, and ginger.

Leafy greens are especially important for diabetics because they contain antioxidants and phytonutrients that can aid in the reduction of inflammation and the improvement of blood sugar control. Apples and oranges are also beneficial because they contain fiber and pectin, which can slow sugar absorption into the bloodstream. Carrots and beets are high in vitamins and minerals, and they can help improve heart health. Tomatoes, cucumbers, and celery are also high in fiber and water, which can aid in digestion. Finally, ginger is an excellent addition to your juice because it aids in the reduction of inflammation and the improvement of circulation.

By incorporating these fruits and vegetables into your juicing routine, you can get a healthy dose of vitamins, minerals, and other nutrients while also helping to regulate your blood sugar levels and improve your overall health.

## Benefits of Juicing Fruits and Vegetables for Diabetes

**1. Nutritious:** Fruits and vegetables are high in vitamins, minerals, fiber, and antioxidants, all of which are beneficial to overall health. The fiber in fruits and vegetables slows the absorption of sugar in the blood, which aids in blood sugar regulation.

**2. Low in Calories:** Fruits and vegetables are naturally low in calories, which can help diabetics manage their weight better.

**3. Low in Sugar:** Although many fruits and vegetables contain naturally occurring sugars, they are typically much lower in sugar content than added sugars found in processed foods.

**4. High in Vitamins and Minerals:** Fruits and vegetables are high in vitamins and minerals that are essential for good health.

**5. Fiber:** Fiber slows digestion and sugar absorption in the blood, which helps to regulate blood sugar levels.

**6. Low on the Glycemic Index:** Fruits and vegetables have a low glycemic index, which means they won't cause blood sugar spikes.

**7. Fruits and vegetables**: provide natural sweetness without the added sugars found in processed foods. This can assist diabetics in better managing their blood sugar levels.

**8. Convenience**: Juicing fruits and vegetables is a quick and easy way to get your daily fruit and vegetable servings.

**9. Variety**: Juicing allows people to combine various fruits and vegetables to obtain a wide range of nutrients.

**10. Delicious**: Juicing can help make fruits and vegetables more appealing and help you incorporate them into your diet in a tasty way.

Fruits and vegetables are good for diabetics because they are high in vitamins and minerals, low in calories and sugar, and high in fiber, which helps regulate blood sugar levels. In conclusion, fruits and vegetables are a healthy choice for diabetics because they are naturally low in calories, sugar, and fat while also providing essential vitamins and minerals.

Fruits and Vegetables for Juicing with Diabetes" refers to a dietary approach in which people with diabetes consume fruits and vegetables in liquid form, obtained through the use of a juicer or a blender.

Juicing fruits and vegetables allows for easy and quick nutrient absorption, which can provide several health benefits for people with diabetes.

When fruits and vegetables are juiced, their fiber content is typically reduced, which can lead to a faster absorption of the juice's natural sugars. This can result in a faster rise in blood sugar levels, which may not be ideal for diabetics. Choosing low-glycemic index fruits and vegetables, as well as adding fiber-rich foods like nuts and seeds to juice, can help mitigate this effect.

Furthermore, juicing can help people with diabetes consume a wider variety of fruits and vegetables than they might otherwise be able to due to limitations such as taste preferences, digestion issues, or time constraints. This can result in a more nutrient-dense diet high in vitamins, minerals, and antioxidants, all of which are beneficial to overall health and blood sugar control.

While juicing can provide health benefits for people with diabetes, it should not be used as the sole source of fruits and vegetables in a balanced diet.

It's also important to eat whole fruits and vegetables because they contain fiber and other important nutrients that juice lacks. Furthermore, because individual needs vary, it is critical to consult with a healthcare provider to determine the best dietary approach for managing diabetes.

Juicing can be a convenient way for diabetics to consume fruits and vegetables on the go, particularly if they have a busy schedule or limited access to fresh produce.

Juicing allows diabetics to experiment with different fruit and vegetable combinations, which can help them discover new flavors and nutrients.

When juicing, choose low-sugar fruits and vegetables like leafy greens, cucumber, and berries and avoid adding extra sugar or sweeteners to the juice.

Drinking juice can cause a more rapid spike in blood sugar levels than eating whole fruits and vegetables, so blood sugar levels should be monitored and insulin or other medications adjusted as needed.

Juicing should not be used in place of a varied diet that includes lean proteins, healthy fats, and complex carbohydrates.

To prevent the growth of harmful bacteria, it is critical to thoroughly clean and sanitize the juicer or blender after each use.

Juicing can be costly, so before beginning a juicing regimen, consider the cost of purchasing fresh produce as well as investing in a juicer or blender. Many people, however, believe that the health benefits of juicing are worth the cost.

Juicing should not be used in place of whole fruits and vegetables in a balanced diet. Juicing can be a great way to supplement a healthy diet, but it's also important to eat a variety of whole foods to ensure that your body gets all of the nutrients it requires. Additionally, before making any significant changes to your diet, especially if you have diabetes, consult with a healthcare provider.

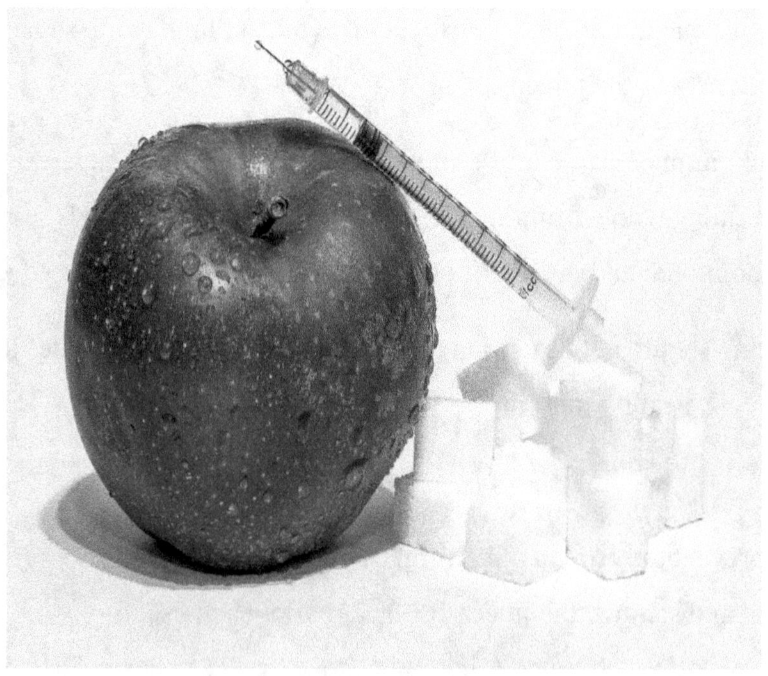

# CHAPTER SIX

## Juicing and Weight Management

Juicing has become a popular weight-loss method for good reason. Juicing can help you lose weight by providing essential nutrients to your body, decreasing cravings for unhealthy foods, and promoting healthy digestion. However, before incorporating juicing into your weight loss plan, it is critical to understand the benefits and potential drawbacks.

To begin with, juicing can be a great way to increase your intake of fruits and vegetables. Fruits and vegetables are high in essential nutrients such as vitamins, minerals, and fiber, which can aid in healthy weight management. Juicing allows you to consume more fruits and vegetables than you would be able to eat whole, allowing you to get more nutrients in each serving.

Juicing can help to reduce cravings for unhealthy foods in addition to providing essential nutrients. When you drink a high-nutrient juice, your body feels more satisfied and is less likely to crave sugary or high-fat foods. This can assist you in avoiding overeating and remaining on track with your weight-loss objectives.

Another advantage of juicing is that it can help with digestion. When you drink juice, you're getting a concentrated source of nutrients that your body can easily absorb. This can aid in the promotion of healthy digestion and the overall health of your digestive system. When your digestive system is working properly, your body is better able to absorb and utilize the nutrients from the foods you eat, which can help you maintain a healthy weight.

It is important to note, however, that juicing should not be used in place of whole fruits and vegetables. Whole fruits and vegetables contain significant amounts of dietary fiber, which can aid in blood sugar regulation and promote feelings of fullness. Juices without this fiber can cause a rapid spike in blood sugar levels, leading to cravings and overeating.

If you are not careful, juicing can be high in calories. Some juices contain added sugars or other high-calorie ingredients that, if consumed in excess, can contribute to weight gain. Juices that are low in sugar and calories should be consumed in moderation as part of a well-balanced diet. When done correctly, juicing can be an effective way to aid in weight loss. You can increase your intake of essential nutrients, reduce cravings for unhealthy foods, and promote healthy digestion by incorporating nutrient-rich juices into your diet.

However, it is important to remember that juicing should not be used in place of whole fruits and vegetables and that low-sugar, low-calorie juices should be consumed in moderation as part of a balanced diet. Juicing is an excellent way to aid in weight management. You can get a concentrated dose of the nutrients your body requires by juicing fruits and vegetables without consuming too many calories. Juicing can help you feel fuller for longer periods of time and provide you with more energy throughout the day. It can also aid in the reduction of cravings and the promotion of healthy eating habits.

Juicing is an excellent way to meet your daily vitamin and mineral requirements. Fruits and vegetables contain essential nutrients such as vitamins A, C, and E, as well as minerals such as calcium and iron. Juicing provides you with the nutrients you need in a concentrated form without consuming a lot of calories.

Juicing can also help your body detoxify and flush out toxins. Juicing can help you lose weight and live a healthier lifestyle. Juicing is an excellent way to get a lot of vitamins and nutrients without consuming a lot of calories. Drinking fresh juice can help you feel fuller longer and avoid overeating. Juicing can also be an excellent way to detoxify the body, as many juices contain vitamins, minerals, antioxidants, and other beneficial compounds that can aid in the removal of toxins and promote overall health. Furthermore, because many juices are mostly water, juicing can be a great way to keep your body hydrated. Finally, juicing is a great way to increase your intake of fruits and vegetables, which can provide valuable nutrients and fiber that can aid in weight loss.

To get the most out of juicing for weight loss, keep in mind that it should not be used in place of whole fruits and vegetables. Although juicing can provide important vitamins, minerals, and other beneficial compounds, it is also important to get these nutrients from whole fruits and vegetables. Furthermore, the amount of added sugars and other ingredients that may be added to some juices should be monitored, as these can add unnecessary calories to your diet.

Juicing can also aid in the maintenance of a healthy weight. You can fill up on healthy nutrients without consuming too many calories by eating the right amount of fruits and vegetables. Juicing can also aid in the reduction of cravings, which can result in overeating and unhealthy snacking. Juicing can also help you stay active and burn calories by boosting your energy levels.

juicing is an excellent way to aid in weight management. It can help to provide your body with the essential nutrients it requires while also reducing cravings, increasing energy levels, and aiding in detoxification. Juicing is an excellent way to get the nutrients you require while maintaining a healthy weight.

Juicing and weight loss are inextricably linked, as juicing can be used to help manage weight and promote overall health.

The process of extracting juice from fresh fruits and vegetables is known as juicing. This juice can then be drunk straight or used to make smoothies, shakes, and other healthy recipes.

Juicing can help with weight loss because it is a quick and easy way to get a variety of vitamins, minerals, and phytonutrients into your diet. Juice can also help you feel fuller, making it easier to eat less and stick to your calorie goals.

Drinking freshly squeezed juice can also help reduce your desire for unhealthy snacks. It can be a healthy substitute for processed and sugary snacks, which can derail your diet.

Juicing can help with weight management by increasing your metabolism in addition to providing nutritional benefits. Fresh fruits and vegetables contain enzymes that aid in the breakdown and digestion of food. This can assist you in burning more calories and losing weight more quickly.

Juicing can be an excellent way to consume the recommended daily servings of fruits and vegetables. Fruits and vegetables are an important part of any well-balanced diet and can aid in weight loss. Juicing can be extracted from fruits and vegetables. It is frequently used as part of a healthy diet for weight loss. Juicing can aid in weight loss by providing essential vitamins, minerals, and antioxidants found in fruits and vegetables. It can also assist people in making healthier food choices by providing more nutritious snacks and meals. Juicing, when done correctly, can be an excellent way to stay healthy and maintain a healthy weight.

Weight management is the process of controlling one's weight through diet and exercise. Eating a well-balanced diet rich in fruits and vegetables, as well as regular exercise, are critical components of successful weight management. Maintaining a healthy weight can lower your risk of developing chronic illnesses like diabetes, heart disease, and cancer. It can also help with mood, energy levels, and overall quality of life.

Juicing and weight loss go hand in hand. Juicing can provide essential nutrients while also assisting people in making healthier food choices. It can also be used as a snack or meal replacement to help you lose weight by lowering your calorie intake. Juicing, when combined with regular exercise, can help people achieve and maintain a healthy weight.

Overall, juicing can be an excellent way to aid in weight loss. Juicing can provide important vitamins, minerals, and other beneficial compounds while also keeping you hydrated and full.

It can also help you increase your intake of fruits and vegetables, which can provide important nutrients and fiber. However, in order to achieve long-term weight management results, juicing should be used in conjunction with a healthy, balanced diet and regular exercise.

## How to go about Juicing and Weight Management

Juicing and weight loss are inextricably linked. Juicing can be a great way to get extra nutrients, vitamins, minerals, and antioxidants while also helping you maintain a healthy weight. Here are some pointers for juicing and weight loss:

**1. Select the Right Juices**: When juicing for weight loss, it is critical to select juices that are low in calories and high in nutrients. Look for juices that are high in fiber, vitamins, minerals, and antioxidants and are made from fruits and vegetables. Juices high in sugar or artificial sweeteners should be avoided because they can quickly add up in calories and sabotage your weight loss efforts.

**2. Portion Control:** It is critical to practice portion control when juicing for weight loss. Begin with smaller servings and gradually increase your juice consumption over time.

**3. Increase Physical Activity:** While juicing can assist you in maintaining a healthy weight, it is also important to combine it with physical activity. Get at least 30 minutes of physical activity per day to help you reach your weight-loss goals.

**4. Drink Enough Water:** Water is important for weight loss. Make a concerted effort to consume plenty of water..

**5. Avoid Unhealthy Foods:** While juicing can help you get more nutrients, it is still important to avoid unhealthy foods. Consuming processed foods, refined sugars, and unhealthy fats can quickly undermine your weight-loss efforts.

**6. Eat a Balanced Diet:** Eating a balanced diet will assist you in meeting your weight management objectives. Consume plenty of fruits and vegetables, lean proteins, whole grains, and healthy fats.

You can help maintain a healthy weight and get all the nutrients your body requires by following these juicing and weight management tips.

In addition to your juices, drink water throughout the day to help you stay hydrated and reach your weight-loss goals.

# benefits of Juicing and Weight Management

**1. Increased nutrient intake**: Juicing allows you to consume more nutrients from fruits and vegetables. This can help you meet your daily vitamin and mineral requirements, which can aid in weight management.

**2. Lower calorie intake**: Juicing removes the majority of the fiber from fruits and vegetables, lowering the calorie content. This makes it easier to follow a low-calorie diet, which can aid in weight loss.

**3. Appetite control:** Juicing can help with weight management by reducing cravings and hunger.

**4. Improved digestion:** Juicing aids in the breakdown of fruit and vegetable cell walls, making it easier for your body to digest and absorb nutrients. This helps to improve digestion, which can aid in weight loss.

**5. Detoxification:** Juicing aids in the removal of toxins from the body, which can reduce inflammation and bloating. This can aid in weight loss.

**6. Increased energy levels**: Juicing can help you feel more energized, which can motivate you to be more active and exercise more. This can help with weight loss.

Juicing can help to improve mood and reduce stress, which can help to reduce emotional eating. This can help with weight loss.

Overall, juicing can be an effective weight-loss tool. It can aid in increasing nutrient intake, decreasing calorie intake, controlling appetite, improving digestion, detoxifying the body, increasing energy levels, and improving mood. All of these advantages can contribute to healthy weight management.

It is important to note, however, that juicing should not be used in place of healthy eating and exercise. It should be used as an additional tool for weight management and should not be used in place of a healthy diet and regular exercise.

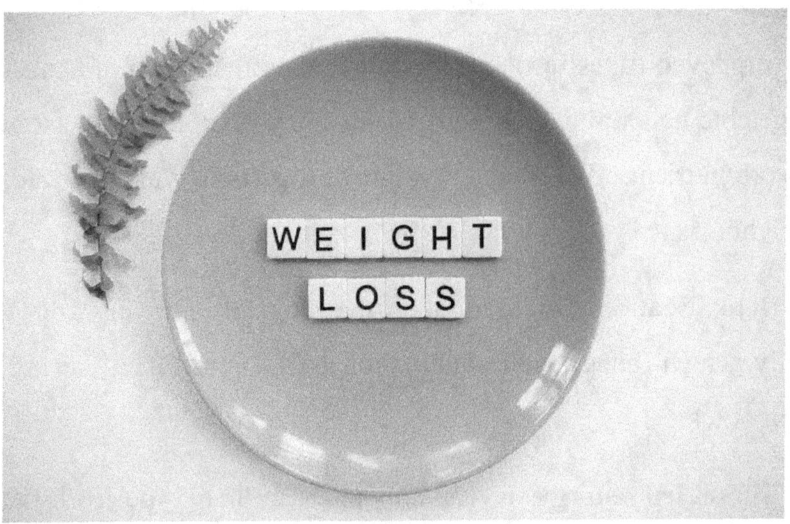

# CHAPTER SEVEN

## Juicing and Exercise

Exercise and juicing are two popular health practices that have grown in popularity in recent years. While each of these practices has distinct advantages, combining them can significantly improve your health and wellness. In this article, we'll look at the benefits of juicing and exercise, how they work together to improve your health, and how to effectively incorporate them into your daily routine.

Exercise is essential for both physical and mental health.. Regular exercise helps to strengthen your muscles, bones, and joints, as well as improve your cardiovascular health, weight management, stress management, and cognitive function. Endorphins are natural mood-boosting chemicals released during exercise that can help reduce stress and anxiety while also improving mental clarity.

When juicing and exercise are combined, they can create a powerful synergy that can significantly improve your overall health and well-being. Here's how it's done:

**Improved Nutrient Absorption:** By drinking fresh juice before or after exercise, you can give your body a concentrated dose of nutrients that are easily absorbed and utilized. This can help you increase your energy and endurance, allowing you to exercise for longer periods of time.

**Improved Hydration**: Drinking fresh juice is a great way to stay hydrated, which is essential for peak exercise performance. When you exercise, you lose water through sweat, which must be replaced in order to avoid dehydration.

**Reduced Inflammation:** Anti-inflammatory fruits and vegetables, such as ginger, turmeric, and leafy greens, can help to reduce inflammation in the body. This can help with muscle soreness and recovery time after exercise.

**Muscle Recovery:** Drinking fresh juice after exercise can help your body get the nutrients and minerals it needs to support muscle recovery and repair. This can help with muscle soreness and overall muscle function.

Now that we've established the benefits of combining juicing and exercise, here are some pointers on how to do so effectively: To improve nutrient absorption and hydration, drink fresh juice before or after exercise.

To provide your body with the nutrients it needs for optimal health, choose nutrient-dense fruits and vegetables that are high in antioxidants, vitamins, and minerals.

Experiment with different juice recipes to keep things interesting and to ensure you're getting a diverse range of nutrients. In order to target different muscle groups and promote overall health and wellness, incorporating various forms of exercise such as strength training, cardio, and yoga.

**Improved Digestion:** Fresh juice contains enzymes that aid digestion and nutrient absorption. Regularly drinking fresh juice can help to improve your digestive health, reduce bloating and indigestion, and promote regular bowel movements.

**Mental Clarity:** Exercise is beneficial not only to your physical health, but also to your mental health. Endorphins are natural mood-boosting chemicals released during exercise that can help reduce stress and anxiety while also improving mental clarity.

**Weight Loss:** Juicing and exercise can be a powerful weight loss combination. You can promote fat loss by consuming fresh juice instead of sugary drinks and incorporating regular exercise into your routine.

**Immune System Support:** Fresh juice contains immune-boosting vitamins and antioxidants that can help support your immune system. Exercise also improves immune function by increasing circulation and decreasing inflammation.

**Increased Energy**: You can increase your energy levels and reduce fatigue by providing your body with the necessary nutrients and improving circulation through exercise.

**Better Sleep**: Regular exercise can help to improve sleep quality and reduce insomnia, and certain fruits and vegetables, such as cherries and kale, contain sleep-promoting nutrients that can aid in the regulation of sleep-wake cycles.

When incorporating juicing and exercise into your routine, it is critical to begin slowly and gradually build up your routine. Begin with small changes, such as drinking fresh juice a few times per week or incorporating short walks into your daily routine, and gradually increase the intensity and frequency.

Remember to listen to your body and make necessary adjustments. Before making significant changes to your diet or exercise routine, consult with a healthcare professional, especially if you have any underlying health conditions.

## Juice  and exercise how they affect you

**JUICE EFFECT**. Freshly squeezed juice can provide your body with essential vitamins and minerals that are necessary for good health. Drinking juice helps you stay hydrated throughout the day, which is important for maintaining optimal bodily functions.

**Increases immunity:** Many fruits and vegetables used in juices are high in antioxidants, which can help boost your immune system and keep you healthy. Juices can help digestion by promoting the growth of healthy gut bacteria and alleviating constipation. Drinking juice can help you feel fuller for longer, lowering your overall calorie intake and promoting weight loss.

Exercise can help strengthen your heart and improve circulation, lowering your risk of heart disease and other cardiovascular problems.

**Muscle:** can be built and maintained through regular exercise, which is important for overall strength and mobility.

Exercise is a great way to relieve stress and anxiety because it causes the release of endorphins, which promote feelings of well-being.

**Improves sleep quality**: Exercise can help you sleep better and feel more rested and alert during the day.

**Boosts mood and energy**: Regular exercise can help you feel more motivated and productive throughout the day by improving your mood and energy levels.

Walking, running, and weightlifting are all exercises that can help strengthen bones and lower the risk of osteoporosis. Regular exercise can help you maintain muscle mass, flexibility, and balance as you age, lowering your risk of falls and other age-related injuries.

Exercise can help improve immune function by increasing the production of white blood cells, which can aid in the fight against infections and diseases. Regular exercise, according to some studies, can improve fertility in both men and women by regulating hormones and promoting healthy blood flow.

Improves physical fitness, body image, and overall well-being: Regular exercise can help boost self-confidence and self-esteem by improving physical fitness, body image, and overall well-being.

## Some exercises you can practice while incorporating juicing into your routine

**Cardiovascular Exercise:** Cardiovascular exercise, such as running, cycling, swimming, or brisk walking, is an excellent way to improve cardiovascular health, increase energy, and burn calories. Fresh juice can be consumed before or after a cardio workout to provide your body with the necessary nutrients and hydration.

**Strength Training:** Weight lifting and resistance band workouts, for example, can help you build muscle mass, improve bone density, and boost your metabolism. Consuming fresh juice after a strength training workout can supply your body with the nutrients and minerals it requires to support muscle recovery and repair.

**Yoga or Pilates:** Yoga and Pilates are both low-impact exercises that can help you improve your flexibility, balance, and core strength. Fresh juice consumed before or after your yoga or Pilates session can help to improve hydration and provide your body with the nutrients it requires.

**High-Intensity Interval Training**: HIIT workouts consist of short bursts of high-intensity exercise followed by rest periods. These workouts are great for losing weight, improving cardiovascular health, and increasing endurance. You can drink fresh juice before or after your HIIT workout to boost energy and aid in muscle recovery.

Hiking, cycling, and kayaking are examples of outdoor activities that can provide a fun and enjoyable way to exercise while taking in the beauty of nature. Fresh juice consumed before or after an outdoor activity can help to improve hydration and provide your body with the nutrients it requires.

Keep in mind that the type of exercise you choose is determined by your fitness level, preferences, and goals. It is critical to listen to your body and select exercises that you enjoy and can maintain over time. You can reap the many benefits of both practices and achieve your health and fitness goals by incorporating fresh juice into your exercise routine.

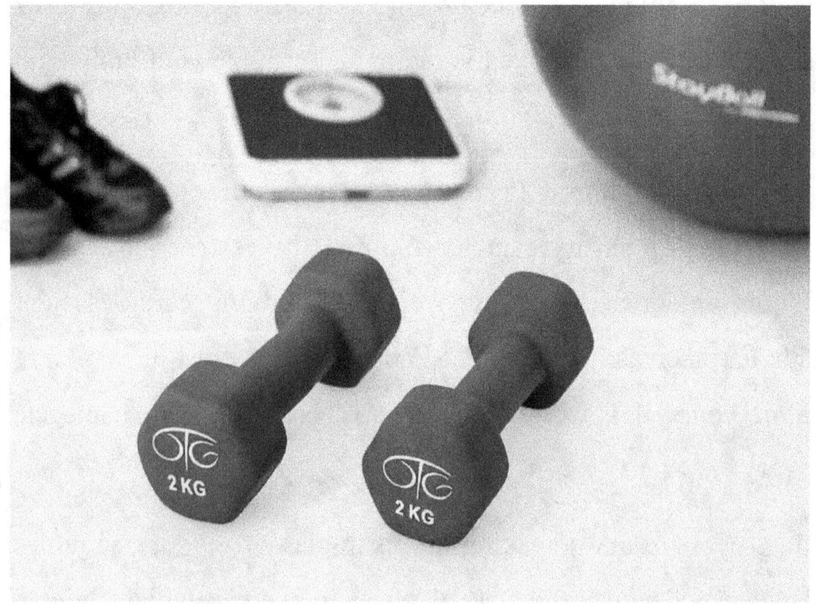

# CHAPTER EIGHT

## Benefits of Juicing to Manage Diabetes

Nutrition is critical for people with type 2 diabetes overall health. They must monitor what they eat and drink at each meal because both can have a significant impact on their blood sugar levels and how they feel.

If you're trying to control your blood glucose levels, sticking to a healthy eating plan may entail giving up some of your favorite treats. Juice drinks, for example, are generally not recommended for people with type 2 diabetes due to their high sugar content. But that doesn't mean you can't enjoy a refreshing glass of orange juice every now and then.

This article will discuss why drinking juice may be harmful to people with type 2 diabetes, as well as the best juice drinks for people with diabetes. Finally, we'll give you recipes and other healthy tips to ensure you're drinking the juice drinks safely.

A glass of juice is often taken for granted by people who do not have type 2 diabetes. This may not be the best option for people with type 2 diabetes.

Diabetes affects how a person's body converts the food they consume into energy. When you eat something, for example, the sugar in the food is broken down and released into your bloodstream. As blood sugar levels rise, the pancreas releases insulin, which allows blood sugar to enter cells and be used for energy.

If you have diabetes, your body most likely does not produce enough insulin or cannot use the insulin that it does produce to pull blood sugar into cells for energy. High blood glucose levels and other complications result if blood glucose levels are not brought down to healthy levels.

Fruits are high in fiber, which is an important nutrient because it slows the rate of glucose or sugar absorption from the gastrointestinal tract. When it comes to fruit juices, however, most of the fiber is removed during the juicing process, leaving mostly sugar, which, when consumed, can cause a rapid and high spike in blood glucose level.

While most people will have no problems drinking juice, those with diabetes may be unable to do so due to the risks associated with rapid increases in blood sugar levels in diabetics.

# These are the benefits and drawbacks of drinking juice for type 2 diabetes.

Many people enjoy drinking juice to start their day. Juices, whether you have diabetes or not, should be consumed in moderation. Fruit juices are high in calories per serving, have more sugar than is recommended for daily consumption, and lack fiber that whole fruits do.

So, why do people continue to reach for a glass of juice as a healthy snack? This is frequently because, depending on the fruit juice, it can provide some benefits, and those with type 2 diabetes may be able to reap some of these benefits.

Fruit juice, for example, is an excellent source of vitamin C, a nutrient required for development, body tissue repair, and growth. It also aids in the formation of collagen and iron absorption, as well as the proper functioning of the immune system.

Consuming vegetables and fruit juices has been linked to a lower incidence of numerous chronic diseases such as cardiovascular disease, cancer, and neurodegenerative diseases, according to studies1. As a result, this study indicates that fruits and vegetable juices can benefit the vascular system and heart.

One hundred percent fruit juice, for example, contains bioactive compounds with antioxidant activity that can improve antioxidant status and blood lipid levels. Nonetheless, while a cup of orange juice can meet a person's daily vitamin C requirement, eating fruits and vegetables should be the preferred method of obtaining this nutrient, especially given all of the disadvantages of drinking juice. Those with type 2 diabetes, for example, who consume too many juice drinks may experience weight gain and hyperglycemia.

Hyperglycemia, or a rapid rise in blood sugar levels, can lead to a number of potentially fatal conditions, including:

1) hyperosmolar hyperglycemic state resulting in severe dehydration

2) Diabetic ketoacidosis, which can result in coma.

Chronic hyperglycemia can harm organs such as the eyes, kidneys, nerves, and blood vessels. Damage to these blood vessels can also increase your chances of having a stroke or having a heart attack, as well as delaying wound healing. This is also why many people choose to obtain these benefits through juices. It is frequently a faster and more compact way for them to meet their daily vitamin, mineral, and antioxidant recommendations, which can have a significant impact on their health.

If you drink juice, you should be aware of hyperglycemia symptoms such as tiredness, blurred vision, increased thirst, dry mouth, and a general feeling of being ill.

## Juices that are beneficial for type 2 diabetes

Although people with type 2 diabetes are often advised to drink low-calorie, low-sugar drinks, they can also drink juices. Consider the following examples:

## Juice from fruits

While it is generally recommended to avoid fruit juices due to their high sugar content, juices with lower sugar content should be consumed if necessary.

This means choosing 100% natural juices with no added sugars and avoiding pineapple or mango juices. These fruit juices frequently contain a significant amount of sugar. Choose unsweetened lemon or grapefruit juice instead, which has a lower glycemic index than most other juices.

## Juice from vegetables

Fresh vegetable juices are often better for type 2 diabetes because they have a lower glycemic index and a high amount of antioxidants.

Low glycemic index foods have been shown to help control type 2 diabetes and aid in weight loss.

As a result, those with diabetes should try juices made from kale and spinach, which are excellent at regulating blood sugar levels.

These are the best juices for people with type 2 diabetes.

If grapefruit juice is not your preferred beverage, there are several other juices that may be beneficial to people with type 2 diabetes, including:

**Tomato juice**

Tomato juice is an excellent choice for people with type 2 diabetes. It has been shown to reduce the risk of blood clots, which is a common problem for diabetics due to the increased risk of developing atherosclerosis and cardiovascular issues.

**The juice of pomegranate**

This juice is high in fiber, folate, potassium, and vitamin C. This juice also contains a high concentration of antioxidants. Pomegranate juice is also a good option for diabetics due to its low glycemic index. According to studies2, they are beneficial in controlling diabetes and some of its complications.

**Juice from carrots**

Despite their sweet flavor, carrots can help manage blood glucose levels and, when consumed in moderation, will not spike blood sugar levels.

Carrots also contain a variety of minerals, vitamins, and carotenoids, which act as antioxidants and benefit the body. Despite having a low glycemic index, a 250gm serving of carrot juice contains 23gm of carbohydrates.

Another great juice blend to try is combining a variety of vegetables, such as leafy vegetables, cucumbers, or celery, with various berries. This can provide you with a tasty drink that is high in vitamins and minerals.

Make a note of the berries and include them in your total carbohydrate count.

Healthy Juice Drinking Suggestions

Although drinking juice can be a great way to get some vegetables and fruit into your diet, diabetics must be careful about what is in these juices and how to consume them.

The following healthy tips will help you understand how to incorporate juice into your diet even if you have type 2 diabetes.

Select diabetes-friendly low-sugar beverages.

Certain fruit juices are preferable to others because they do not cause a massive sugar spike. If you must have a juice drink, choose one that is 100% pure and low in natural sugar. Alternatively, if possible, choose a vegetable juice because fresh vegetables have a lower glycemic index.

**Consume juice with your meal**.

Another great way to enjoy a cup of juice is with a meal. While juice can cause a blood sugar spike, combining it with other foods, particularly those high in fiber, healthy fats, or protein, can help prevent it.

**Consume small amounts of juice**

If you feel the need for a glass of juice, limit yourself to four to eight ounces. By keeping the amount low, you can avoid the juice wreaking havoc on your blood sugar levels and having serious consequences.

Take note of the added sugar on the nutrition label.

Another reason why drinking homemade juice is often preferable is that store-bought juices frequently contain several extra ingredients and sweeteners, making an already sugary drink even sweeter.

If you have to drink juice from a store for any reason, make sure to read the nutrition label to find out exactly what is in the juice. Take note of the serving size, calories, and ingredients.

**Concentrate on non-starchy vegetables.**

Non-starchy vegetables are just a few of the food groups that diabetics can eat to satisfy their hunger. Minerals, fiber, vitamins, and phytochemicals abound in these. They also contain fewer calories and carbohydrates, which is essential for a healthy diet.

**Some of the more common non-starchy vegetables to consider including in your juices are:**

Beets

Broccoli

Carrots

Cauliflower

Celery

Leeks

Cucumber

Mushrooms

**When should I consult a dietician?**

Diabetes requires you to be cautious about what you eat and drink.. As a result, your doctor may advise you to consult with a dietician.

A dietician can assist you in developing a healthy eating plan and answering questions about which foods to avoid and which foods to eat to keep your blood sugar levels in check.

These experts can devise a strategy that is tailored to your specific goals, lifestyle, and preferences. They can also help you understand the best portion sizes for you, improve your eating habits, and make the most of the insulin your body produces or receives from medication.

Diabetes patients frequently have unique requirements. While there are no specific rules for their diet, these individuals must keep certain things in mind, especially when managing their blood sugar, such as eating a balanced diet, managing their carbohydrate intake, and checking blood sugar levels on a regular basis.

These factors, however, should not prevent people with type 2 diabetes from enjoying their favorite foods, including fruit juice. It simply means that they must consume their juices in moderation and keep track of how this sweet treat may affect their bodies.

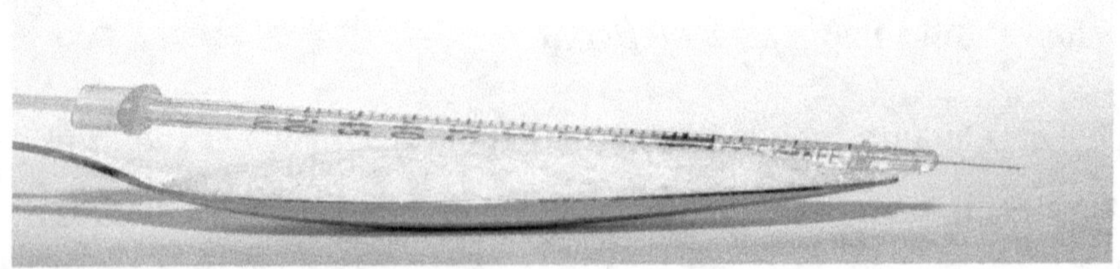

**More benefits of juicing to manage diabetes:**

Provides essential nutrients: Juicing fruits and vegetables is an excellent way to obtain essential nutrients that can aid in diabetes management. Leafy greens, for example, contain vitamins A, C, and K, as well as magnesium and potassium, all of which can help regulate blood sugar levels.

**Lowers inflammation**: Juicing can also help reduce inflammation in the body, which is important for diabetics because high levels of inflammation can make controlling blood sugar levels more difficult. Many fruits and vegetables contain anti-inflammatory compounds such as flavonoids and carotenoids, which can aid in the reduction of inflammation in the body.

Maintaining a healthy weight is important for people with diabetes, and juicing can be a useful tool for achieving and maintaining a healthy weight. Juicing can encourage people to eat more fruits and vegetables, which are low in calories but high in fiber and other important nutrients that can make people feel full and satisfied.

**Juicing may help improve insulin sensitivity**: Insulin resistance is a common problem among people with type 2 diabetes, and it is possible that juicing will help improve insulin sensitivity. Consuming certain fruits and vegetables, such as bitter melon, has been shown in some studies to improve insulin sensitivity and lower blood sugar levels.

Can help reduce the risk of complications: Finally, juicing can help reduce the risk of diabetes complications such as cardiovascular disease. Many fruits and vegetables are high in antioxidants, which can help protect against the damage caused by high blood sugar levels and lower the risk of complications developing over time.

Overall, juicing can be a useful tool for diabetes management if done in moderation and as part of a well-balanced diet. Working with a healthcare provider and a registered dietitian to determine the best approach for your specific needs and health goals is critical.

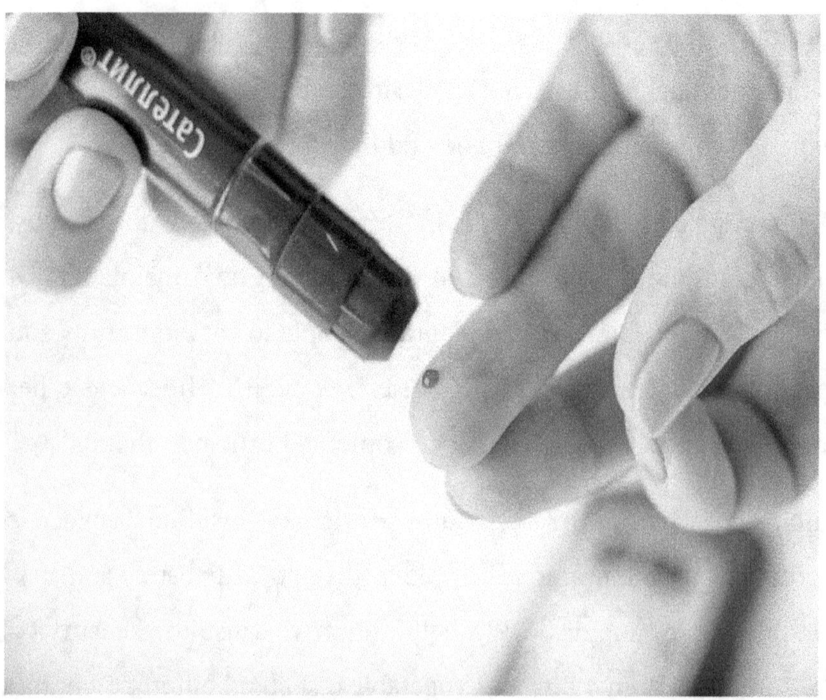

# CHAPTER NINE

## Precautions and Safety Tips for Juicing with Diabetes

Juicing can be a healthy way to include more fruits and vegetables in your diet, but it's important for people with diabetes to take some extra precautions to ensure safety and avoid potential health risks. Here are some things to remember when juicing with diabetes.

Always be prepared to identify yourself as a diabetic in waiting areas, long lines, or areas where having a meal or taking your medication is inconvenient. Always keep glucose tablets or orange juice on hand when traveling.

Never take diabetes medication if you are unsure when your next meal will be. Never take another person's medication. Learn about the possible side effects of your medications.. Know the symptoms of a glycemic attack, whether your blood sugar is low or high. Make a plan with your primary care provider and pharmacist to get refills and avoid having empty prescriptions.

**Personal Hygiene**: Diabetes and physical activities go hand in hand; diabetes control is improved when an individual engages in physical activities such as walking, running, gardening, swimming, and so on.

Eat more vegetables and fruits, and drink sugar-free water instead of sugary drinks. Using a home glucose tester, keep a diary of your readings and provide a summary to your care provider.

**Skincare**: is critical. Choose a month to perform a full skin examination. Pay attention to limbs, toes, or areas that you may overlook on a daily basis. Lubricate dry skin well and pat dry areas with constant moisture, pubic are essential. If you use needles, avoid using dirty needles, reusing needles, and sharing needles. Needles should be disposed of in a container that is not accessible to children or for removal. Inquire with your pharmacy about proper disposal.

**Consult your doctor about the following**: Before incorporating juicing into your diet, consult with your healthcare provider to ensure it is safe for you. They may have specific recommendations or restrictions based on your individual health needs.

**Choose fruits and vegetables with low glycemic indexes**: High-glycemic fruits and vegetables can cause a dangerous spike in blood sugar levels, which can be dangerous for diabetics. Low-glycemic fruits and vegetables, such as kale, spinach, cucumber, celery, and berries, should be consumed.

**Add no sugar or sweeteners:** Many juicing recipes call for added sugar or sweeteners, which can cause blood sugar levels to spike. Choose naturally sweet fruits and vegetables such as carrots or beets instead.

**Monitor your blood sugar levels:** Because juicing can affect your blood sugar levels, it's critical to check them on a regular basis, especially after trying a new juice recipe.

While juicing can be a healthy way to consume more fruits and vegetables, it is important to be mindful of portion sizes. Too much juice consumed at once can result in a rapid rise in blood sugar levels.

**Properly store juice**: Freshly made juice can spoil quickly and develop harmful bacteria, so it is critical to store it properly. Refrigerate your juice in an airtight container and consume it within 24 hours.

**Take a look at the entire fruit:** Juicing removes fiber from fruits and vegetables, which can result in faster sugar absorption in the bloodstream. Consider including whole fruits and vegetables in your diet to slow sugar absorption and provide more nutrients and fiber.

**Begin slowly**: If you're new to juicing, start with small amounts and gradually increase your juice consumption.

**Blood sugar levels should be checked**: Never drink juice on an empty stomach or without first checking your blood sugar levels.

**Fruits and vegetables with low sugar content:** Reduce your intake of high-sugar fruits such as grapes, bananas, pineapple, and mango, and replace them with low-sugar vegetables such as kale, spinach, and celery.

**Count carbs**: Keep track of how many carbs you consume in your juice.

**Juice with meals:** Juice with meals can help regulate your blood sugar levels. When purchasing pre-made juices, make sure to read the labels for added sugars.

**Consult your doctor**: Consult your doctor about your juicing plans to ensure that it is safe for you to consume.

**Stick to fresh juices:** Make your own juices from fresh fruits and vegetables whenever possible.

**Consider moderation**: Juicing should not be used in place of a well-balanced diet. Consume juice sparingly and ensure that you get enough key nutrients from other sources.

**Examine your tools**: Clean your juicer on a regular basis to prevent bacteria from growing.

**Consult your doctor:** Before beginning any new diet or exercise program, consult with your doctor to ensure that it is safe for you.

**Keep an eye on your blood sugar levels**: Because juicing can cause rapid changes in your blood sugar levels, it's critical to keep an eye on them.

**Choose low-glycemic fruits and vegetables**: When juicing, low-glycemic fruits and vegetables such as apples, berries, carrots, and leafy greens are best.

**Include protein**: A source of lean protein, such as Greek yogurt, cottage cheese, or almond butter, can help slow the absorption of sugar. Juicing can be a great way to get your daily servings of fruits and vegetables, but it's important to keep portion sizes in mind to avoid consuming too much sugar.

**Drink slowly:** To avoid a blood sugar spike, drink your juice slowly to allow your body to absorb the nutrients more gradually.

**Avoid added sugar:** Juice with added sugar can quickly raise blood sugar levels. Read labels and avoid added sugars.

**Monitor your carbohydrate intake:** Because juicing can be high in carbohydrates, it's important to keep track of your intake and adjust as needed.

Avoid buying juice from the store: Juices purchased in stores are frequently high in added sugars and other unhealthy ingredients. Stick to freshly made juice at home to stay healthy.

**Consult a dietitian:** If you're new to juicing, it's a good idea to consult a dietitian to learn which juices are best for diabetes.

## 5 tips for taking control and cautions with diabetes

1: **Get rid of excess weight**. Diabetes is reduced by losing weight. Participants in one large study reduced their risk of developing diabetes by nearly 60% after losing 7% of their body weight through changes in exercise and diet. To prevent disease progression, the American Diabetes Association recommends that people with prediabetes lose 7% to 10% of their body weight. More weight loss will result in even greater advantages. Determine your weight-loss target based on your current body weight. Discuss with your doctor realistic short-term goals and expectations, such as losing 1 to 2 pounds per week.

2. **Increase your physical activity.** Regular physical activity has numerous advantages. You can benefit from exercise in the following ways: Reduce your weight and Reduce your blood sugar levels

Improve your insulin sensitivity, which will help you keep your blood sugar within a normal range. Most adults' weight loss and maintenance goals include the following: Aerobic activity. Aim for 30 minutes or more of moderate to vigorous aerobic exercise on most days, for a total of at least 150 minutes per week, such as brisk walking, swimming, biking, or running.

Resistance training. Resistance exercise at least twice a week improves your strength, balance, and overall ability to live an active lifestyle. Resistance exercises include weightlifting, yoga, and calisthenics. Inactivity is limited. To help control blood sugar levels, long periods of inactivity, such as sitting at a computer, can be broken up Take a few minutes every 30 minutes to stand, walk around, or do something light.

**3. Consume nutritious plant foods:** Plants supplement your diet with vitamins, minerals, and carbohydrates. Carbohydrates include sugars and starches, which serve as energy sources for your body, as well as fiber. The portion of plant foods that your body is unable to digest or absorb is referred to as dietary fiber. Fiber-rich foods help people lose weight and reduce their risk of diabetes. Consume a variety of fiber-rich, healthy foods, such as:

Fruits such as tomatoes, peppers, and tree fruit

Nonstarchy vegetables include leafy greens, broccoli, and cauliflower. Legumes include beans, chickpeas, and lentils.

Whole grains like whole wheat pasta and bread, whole grain rice, whole oats, and quinoa

Fiber has the following advantages:

Slowing sugar absorption and lowering blood sugar levels Interfering with dietary fat and cholesterol absorption

Managing other risk factors for heart disease, such as high blood pressure and inflammation Because fiber-rich foods are more filling and energy-dense, they can help you eat less.

Avoid "bad carbohydrates," which are high in sugar with little fiber or nutrients: white bread and pastries, white flour pasta, fruit juices, and processed foods containing sugar or high-fructose corn syrup.

**4. Consume healthy fats:** Fatty foods contain a lot of calories and should be consumed in moderation. Eat a variety of foods high in unsaturated fats, also known as "good fats," to aid in weight loss and management. Unsaturated fats, both monounsaturated and polyunsaturated, support heart and vascular health. Nuts and seeds include almonds, peanuts, flaxseed, and pumpkin seeds. The term "smartphone" refers to the use of a smartphone to communicate with others.

your diet. Saturated fats can be reduced by eating low-fat dairy products, as well as lean chicken and pork.

**5. Avoid fad diets in favor of healthier alternatives**: Many fad diets, such as the glycemic index, paleo, or keto diets, may aid in weight loss. However, there is little research on the long-term benefits of these diets or their effectiveness in preventing diabetes.

Your dietary goal should be to lose weight and then keep it off in the future. Healthy dietary decisions must therefore include a strategy that can be maintained as a lifelong habit. Making healthy choices that reflect some of your own food preferences and traditions may be beneficial to you in the long run.

Divide your plate is a simple strategy for helping you make good food choices and eat appropriate portion sizes. These three sections of your plate encourage healthy eating: Fruit and nonstarchy vegetables make up half of the diet.

Protein-rich foods, such as legumes, fish, or lean meats, account for one-quarter of the diet. The American Diabetes Association recommends routine screening for type 2 diabetes with diagnostic tests for all adults 45 and older, as well as the following groups:

People under the age of 45 who are overweight or obese and have one or more diabetes risk factors Women who have experienced gestational diabetes Individuals who have been diagnosed with prediabetes Overweight or obese children with a family history of type 2 diabetes or other risk factors

Discuss your diabetes prevention concerns with your doctor. He or she will appreciate your efforts to prevent diabetes and may make additional suggestions based on your medical history or other factors.

Finally, lifestyle modifications can aid in the prevention of type 2 diabetes, the most common form of the disease. Prevention is especially important if you are predisposed to type 2 diabetes due to being overweight or obese, having high cholesterol, or having a family history of the disease. family history of diabetes. If you have prediabetes (high blood sugar that does not meet the criteria for diabetes), lifestyle changes can prevent or delay the onset of disease.

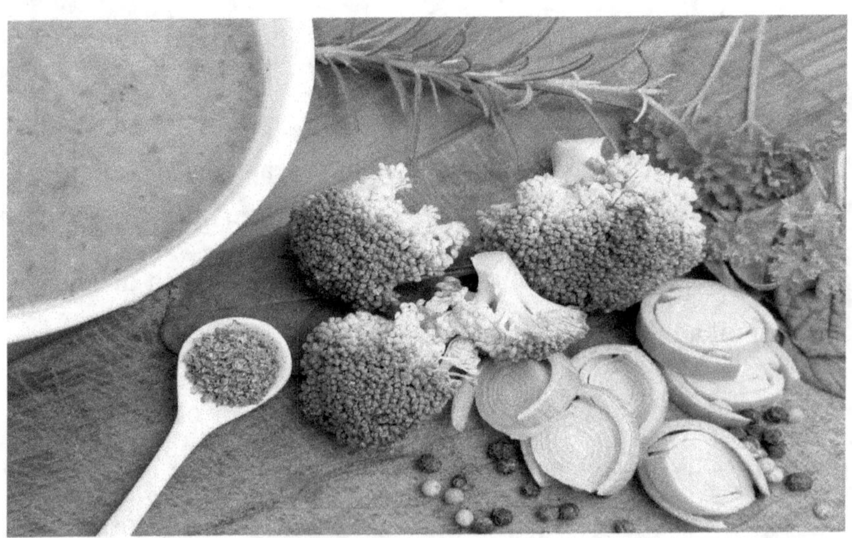

# CHAPTER TEN

## Diabetes fruits and juices to avoid

Diabetes patients must consume a well-balanced diet, exercise regularly, and make lifestyle changes. Fruits are an important part of a well-balanced diet. Certain fruits, on the other hand, can make a diabetic's life hell. Uncontrolled diabetes can lead to a variety of serious complications, including heart disease, kidney disease, blindness, and other complications. These conditions have also been linked to prediabetes. Importantly, certain foods can raise blood sugar and insulin levels as well as promote inflammation, potentially increasing your risk of disease.

## Here are some fruits and juice to avoid

### 1. Beverages with added sugar

If you have diabetes, you should avoid drinking sugary drinks.. For starters, a 12-ounce (354-mL) can of cola contains 38.5 grams of carbs. The same amount of sweetened iced tea and lemonade contain nearly 45 grams of carbs derived entirely from sugar. Furthermore, these drinks are high in fructose, which has been linked to insulin resistance and diabetes. Consuming sugar-sweetened beverages may, in fact, increase the risk of diabetes-related conditions such as fatty liver disease, according to research.

Furthermore, the high fructose content of sugary drinks may cause metabolic changes that promote belly fat as well as potentially harmful cholesterol and triglyceride levels. Consuming 25% of calories from high fructose beverages on a weight-maintenance diet resulted in increased insulin resistance and belly fat, a lower metabolic rate, and worse heart health markers. Consume water, club soda, or unsweetened iced tea instead of sugary beverages to help control blood sugar levels and reduce disease risk.

## 2. Trans fatty acids

Trans fats made from chemicals are extremely harmful. To make unsaturated fatty acids more stable, hydrogen is added to them. Margarine, peanut butter, spreads, creamers, and frozen dinners all contain trans fats. Furthermore, food manufacturers frequently include them in crackers, muffins, and other baked goods to help extend the shelf life of the product.

Trans fats do not directly raise blood sugar levels, but they have been linked to increased inflammation, insulin resistance, and belly fat, as well as lower HDL (good) cholesterol levels and impaired arterial function. While more research is needed to gain a better understanding of the relationship between trans fats and insulin resistance, the links mentioned above are particularly concerning for diabetics, who are at a higher risk of heart disease.

Most countries have banned artificial trans fats, and the Food and Drug Administration (FDA) banned the use of partially hydrogenated oil — the major source of artificial trans fat in the food supply in most processed foods in 2018.

This is not to say that all foods in the United States are now free of trans fats. If a product contains less than 0.5 grams of trans fat per serving, manufacturers are not required to list trans fats on the nutrition facts label. Any product that contains the words "partially hydrogenated" in its ingredient list should be avoided.

**3. Pasta, rice, and white bread**

White bread, rice, and pasta are processed carbohydrate foods. It has been shown that eating bread, bagels, and other refined-flour foods significantly raises blood sugar levels in people with type 1 and type 2 diabetes This reaction is not limited to refined white flour products. Gluten-free pastas were also found to raise blood sugar levels in one study, with rice-based varieties having the greatest effect. Another study discovered that high carbohydrate foods not only raised blood sugar levels but also reduced brain function in people with type 2 diabetes and mental deficits. These processed foods are low in fiber In other studies, replacing low-fiber foods with high-fiber foods was shown to significantly lower blood sugar levels in diabetics. Furthermore, people with diabetes had lower cholesterol levels. Fiber consumption improved gut microbiota, which may have resulted in improved insulin resistance.

## 4. Yogurt with fruit flavors

Diabetes patients may benefit from plain yogurt. Fruit-flavored varieties, on the other hand, are a different story entirely. Flavored yogurts are high in carbohydrates and sugar and are typically made with nonfat or low fat milk. In fact, a 1-cup (245-gram) serving of fruit-flavored yogurt may contain nearly 31 grams of sugar, accounting for nearly 61% of its calories.

Many people believe that frozen yogurt is a healthier alternative to ice cream. It can, however, contain just as much or even more sugar than ice cream.

Rather than choosing high-sugar yogurts, which can cause blood sugar and insulin spikes, choose plain, whole milk yogurt, which contains no sugar and may be beneficial to your appetite, weight control, and gut health.

## 5. Breakfast cereals with added sugar

If you have diabetes, eating cereal can be one of the worst ways to start your day. Despite the health claims on the packaging, most cereals are highly processed and contain far more carbohydrates than most people realize. Furthermore, they contain very little protein, a nutrient that can help you feel full and satisfied while maintaining stable blood sugar levels throughout the day.

Even some "healthy" breakfast cereals are not suitable for diabetics.

A 1/2-cup serving (about 56 grams) of granola, for example, contains 44 grams of carbs, whereas Grape Nuts contain 47 grams. In addition, each serving has no more than 7 grams of protein. Skip most cereals in favor of a protein-based low-carb breakfast to keep blood sugar and hunger under control.

Many breakfast cereals have a high carbohydrate content but a low protein content. Breakfast with a high protein, low carbohydrate content is the best option for diabetes and appetite control.

## 6. Coffee drinks with flavors

Flavored coffee drinks, on the other hand, should be regarded as a liquid dessert rather than a nutritious beverage.

According to research, your brain does not process liquid and solid foods in the same way. When you consume calories, you do not compensate by eating less later, which may result in weight gain.

Carbohydrates are also abundant in flavored coffee drinks.

A 16-ounce (473-mL) Caramel Frappuccino from Starbucks, for example, has 57 grams of carbs, while the sesame-sizef the Blonde Vanilla Latte has 30 grams of carbs. Choose plain coffee or espresso with a tablespoon of heavy cream or half-and-half to keep your blood sugar under control and prevent weight gain.

## 7. Maple syrup, honey, and agave nectar

Diabetics frequently try to limit their intake of white table sugar as well as treats such as candy, cookies, and pie. Other types of sugar, on the other hand, can cause blood sugar spikes. Brown sugar and "natural" sugars like honey, agave nectar, and maple syrup are examples.

Despite the fact that these sweeteners are not highly processed, they contain at least as many carbohydrates as white sugar. In fact, the majority of them contain even more. The carb counts for a 1-tablespoon serving of the following popular sweeteners are listed below:

White sugar: 12.6 g.

17.3 grams of honey.

The amount of agave nectar is 16 grams.

13.4 grams maple syrup.

People with prediabetes experienced similar increases in blood sugar, insulin, and inflammatory markers whether they consumed 1.7 ounces (50 grams) of white sugar or honey, according to one study. Your best bet is to avoid all forms of sugar and instead use natural low carb sweeteners. Although honey, agave nectar, and maple syrup are not as processed as white table sugar, they may have comparable effects on blood sugar, insulin, and inflammatory markers.

## 8. Dried fruit

Fruit is high in several vitamins and minerals, including vitamin C and potassium. When fruit is dried, water is lost, resulting in higher concentrations of these nutrients. Grapes have 27.3 grams of carbs, including 1.4 grams of fiber in one cup (151 grams). In comparison, 1 cup (145 grams) of raisins contains 115 grams of carbs, 5.4 of which are fiber.

As a result, raisins have more than four times the carbs of grapes. Other types of dried fruit are also higher in carbs than their fresh counterparts.

Dried fruits become more concentrated in sugar and may contain up to four times as many carbs as fresh fruits. To maintain optimal blood sugar control, avoid dried fruit and opt for low-sugar fruits.

**9. Snack foods in packages**

Snacking on pretzels, crackers, and other packaged foods is not a good idea. They're typically made with refined flour and contain few nutrients, but they're high in fast-digesting carbs that can quickly raise blood sugar. The carb counts for a 1-ounce (28-gram) serving of some popular snacks are as follows:

20.7 grams of carbs in saltine crackers, including 0.78 grams of fiber. Pretzels contain 22.5 grams of carbohydrates, including 0.95 grams of fiber. Graham crackers have 21.7 grams of carbohydrates, with 0.95 grams of fiber.

In fact, some of these foods may contain even more carbs than the nutrition label indicates. According to one study, snack foods contain 7.7% more carbs than the label claims.

If you get hungry between meals, eat nuts or a few low carb vegetables with an ounce of cheese.

Packaged snacks are often highly processed foods made from refined flour, which can quickly raise blood sugar levels.

## 10. Fruit juice

Although fruit juice is commonly regarded as a healthy beverage, its blood sugar effects are similar to those of sodas and other sugary drinks.

This applies to both unsweetened 100% fruit juice and juice with added sugar. In some cases, fruit juice contains more sugar and carbohydrates than soda. 8 ounces (250 mL) of soda and apple juice, for example, contain 22 and 24 grams of sugar, respectively. A serving of grape juice contains 35 grams of sugar. is high in fructose. Fructose is the primary cause of insulin resistance, obesity, and heart disease.

A much better option is to drink water with a wedge of lemon, which has less than 1 gram of carbs and is almost calorie-free. Fruit juices have at least the same amount of sugar as sodas. Their high fructose content has been linked to insulin resistance, weight gain, and an increased risk of heart disease.

## 11. French Fries

French fries are a food you should avoid, especially if you have diabetes. Potatoes are relatively high in carbohydrates. A medium potato has 34.8 grams of carbs, 2.4 of which are fiber. However, once peeled and fried in vegetable oil, potatoes may do more than just raise blood sugar levels.

Deep-frying foods have been shown to produce high levels of toxic compounds such as AGEs and aldehydes. These compounds have the potential to cause inflammation and increase the risk of disease.

Indeed, several studies have linked eating french fries and other fried foods on a regular basis to heart disease and cancer.

If you don't want to avoid potatoes entirely, a small serving of sweet potatoes is your best bet. French fries are high in carbs, which raise blood sugar levels, and are fried in unhealthy oils, which may promote inflammation and increase the risk of heart disease and cancer.

In conclusion

Knowing which foods to avoid when you have diabetes can be difficult at times. Your main goals should be to avoid unhealthy fats, liquid sugars, processed grains, and other foods high in refined carbohydrates.

Avoiding foods that raise blood sugar levels and promote insulin resistance can help you stay healthy and lower your risk of future diabetes complications.

Remember to choose a variety of fruits and to consume them in moderation. A registered dietitian or healthcare provider can make more specific recommendations about the types and amounts of fruits that are best for a person's health and diabetes management.

Fruits should also be consumed in moderation and balanced with other healthy foods in their diet. It is best to consult a healthcare provider or a registered dietitian for a personalized diet and nutrition recommendations for diabetes management.

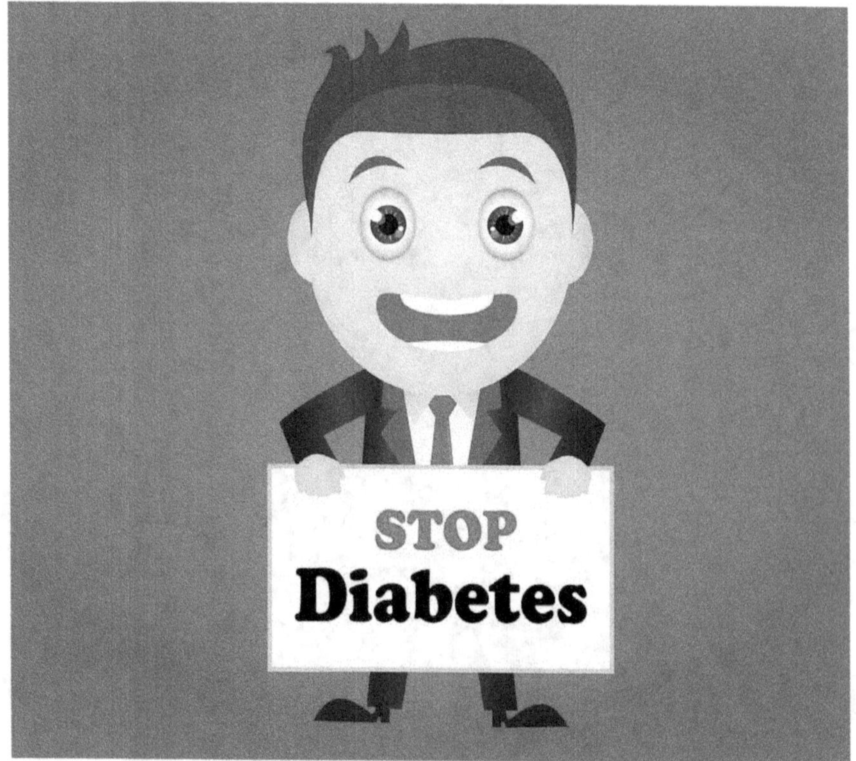

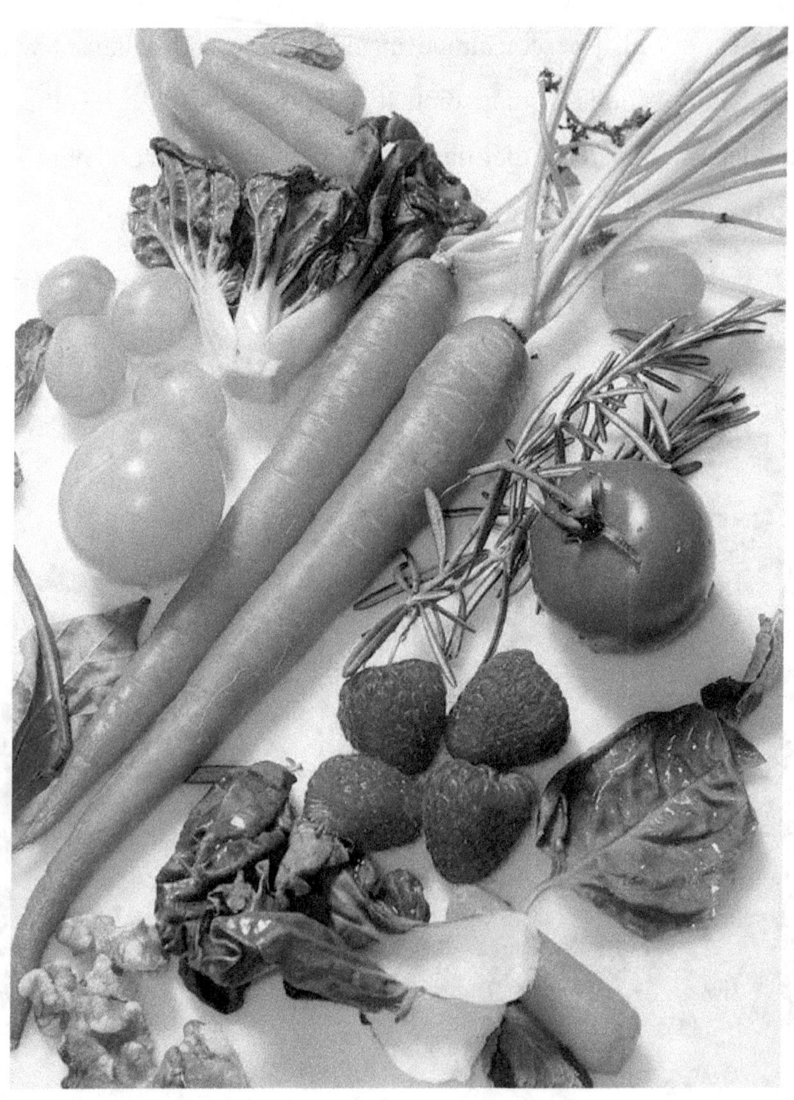

# CONCLUSION

## Conclusion: Integrating Juicing into a Comprehensive Diabetes Management Plan

Conclusion. Diabetes is a serious life-threatening disease that must be constantly monitored and effectively controlled with proper medication and a healthy lifestyle. A healthy lifestyle, regular checkups, and proper medication can help us live a long and healthy life.

Diabetes is a chronic medical condition that necessitates a comprehensive management strategy to keep blood sugar levels under control and complications at bay. While medication, exercise, and a well-balanced diet are the foundations of diabetes management, incorporating juicing into your regimen can be a beneficial way to improve overall health and manage diabetes symptoms. Juicing can be a healthy and enjoyable addition to a diabetes management plan. It can provide important vitamins, minerals, and enzymes that help the body function properly, as well as a way to consume a variety of fruits and vegetables that may be lacking in the diet. Juicing, on the other hand, can cause a rapid rise in blood sugar levels and should be approached with caution. To determine the best approach for each individual, it is critical to consult with a healthcare professional. Juicing can be a safe and enjoyable way to support diabetes management with the right guidance and monitoring. Juicing can be beneficial in the following ways when incorporated into a comprehensive diabetes management plan:

1. Juicing can aid in blood sugar control. Fresh fruits and vegetables contain vitamins, minerals, and phytonutrients that can help balance blood sugar levels and improve insulin sensitivity. Furthermore, the fiber content of fresh fruits and vegetables can slow the absorption of sugar, assisting in the maintenance of stable blood sugar levels.

2. Juicing can supplement the diet with additional nutrients. Fresh fruits and vegetables are high in vitamins and minerals that are essential for good health, such as vitamin A, vitamin C, potassium, and magnesium. Juicing can help to supplement nutrients that may be lacking in a diabetes-focused diet.

3. Juicing can aid in the reduction of inflammation. Fresh fruits and vegetables contain antioxidants and other compounds that can help to reduce inflammation, which is a major factor in the development and progression of diabetes.

4. Juicing can help you relax. Stress is a major cause of diabetes and can make it difficult to manage the condition. Juicing can help reduce stress, which can help with diabetes management.

Individuals can benefit from improved blood sugar control, additional nutrients, reduced inflammation, and reduced stress by incorporating juicing into a comprehensive diabetes management plan. Juicing should be done in moderation because it can cause a spike in blood sugar levels if not done correctly. Diabetes patients should check their blood sugar levels before and after juicing to ensure they are within normal limits. Additionally, before beginning any juicing regimen, it is critical to consult with a healthcare provider. A comprehensive diabetes management plan should also include regular physical activity, a healthy diet, medication adherence, and regular blood sugar monitoring.

Individuals with diabetes can improve their overall health and diabetes management by combining juicing with the other components of a comprehensive diabetes management plan.

In conclusion, juicing can be a beneficial addition to a comprehensive diabetes management plan. It can supply essential nutrients, aid in blood sugar regulation, and promote overall health and well-being.

However, choosing the right ingredients, drinking in moderation, and using juicing as a supplement to a balanced diet are all important. Always consult with your healthcare provider before making major changes to your diabetes management plan.

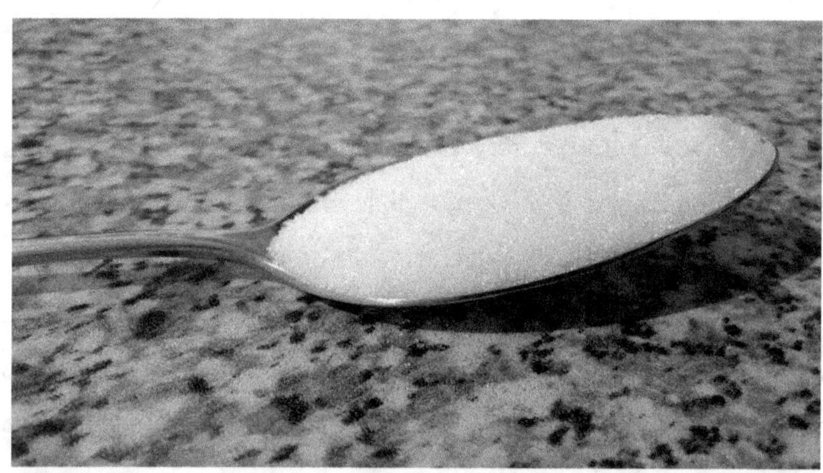

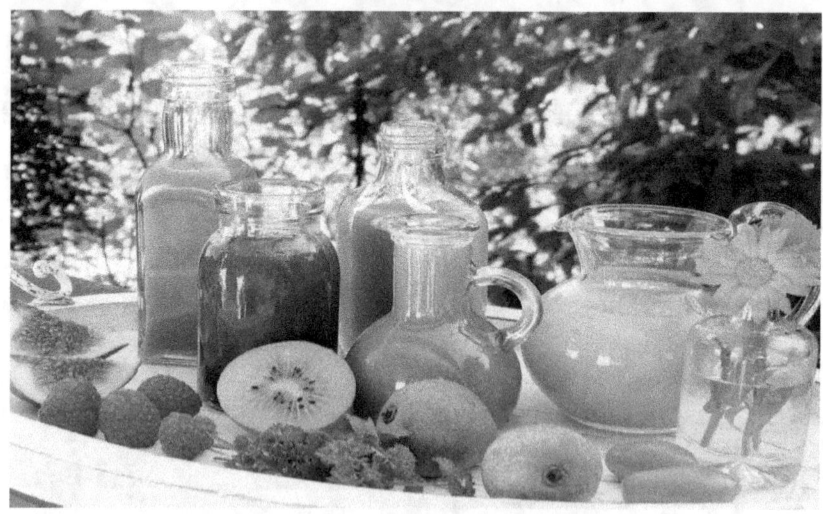

www.ingramcontent.com/pod-product-compliance
Lightning Source LLC
Chambersburg PA
CBHW050812250726
48653CB00006B/2188